Clinician's Guide to Diagnostic Imaging

William R. Reinus
Editor

Clinician's Guide to Diagnostic Imaging

Springer

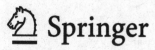

Editor
William R. Reinus, MD, MBA, FACR
Department of Radiology
Temple University Hospital
Philadelphia, PA, USA

ISBN 978-1-4614-8768-5 ISBN 978-1-4614-8769-2 (eBook)
DOI 10.1007/978-1-4614-8769-2
Springer New York Heidelberg Dordrecht London

Library of Congress Control Number: 2013949764

© Springer Science+Business Media New York 2014
This work is subject to copyright. All rights are reserved by the Publisher, whether the whole or part of the material is concerned, specifically the rights of translation, reprinting, reuse of illustrations, recitation, broadcasting, reproduction on microfilms or in any other physical way, and transmission or information storage and retrieval, electronic adaptation, computer software, or by similar or dissimilar methodology now known or hereafter developed. Exempted from this legal reservation are brief excerpts in connection with reviews or scholarly analysis or material supplied specifically for the purpose of being entered and executed on a computer system, for exclusive use by the purchaser of the work. Duplication of this publication or parts thereof is permitted only under the provisions of the Copyright Law of the Publisher's location, in its current version, and permission for use must always be obtained from Springer. Permissions for use may be obtained through RightsLink at the Copyright Clearance Center. Violations are liable to prosecution under the respective Copyright Law.
The use of general descriptive names, registered names, trademarks, service marks, etc. in this publication does not imply, even in the absence of a specific statement, that such names are exempt from the relevant protective laws and regulations and therefore free for general use.
While the advice and information in this book are believed to be true and accurate at the date of publication, neither the authors nor the editors nor the publisher can accept any legal responsibility for any errors or omissions that may be made. The publisher makes no warranty, express or implied, with respect to the material contained herein.

Printed on acid-free paper

Springer is part of Springer Science+Business Media (www.springer.com)

Preface

One of the central principles of patient management is that one should only request studies, whether laboratory tests or imaging examinations, on patients when there is reason to believe that the result will affect patient management. While this may appear as a near truism, it is surprising how often this tenet is not followed. The most common reason that unindicted studies are requested is that the patient wants a test of some sort and the clinician for social, political, economic, and medico-legal reasons feels obligated to oblige. This type of expenditure, though typically wasteful and at times dangerous to the patient, will continue to one degree or another as long as there are doctors and patients. This book will not address this issue other than to advise that under these circumstances clinicians choose the least invasive, dangerous, and costly examination that will suffice.

Instead, the goal of this handbook is to provide best practice guidelines for patients whose management depends on a clinical question that is best approached through imaging. While on the surface the appropriate test to obtain may seem obvious, in this day of a constantly growing and ever enlarging armamentarium of imaging procedures, choosing the correct test at times can be difficult. Compound this with the fact that all imaging procedures are not available at all times or at all institutions or even to all patients because of individual or idiosyncratic contraindications. Thus, imaging management can become a maze. We hope to provide a guide through this maze, indicating first- and second-line imaging examinations for clinicians to use in their daily practice.

Our approach will be by organ system or rather body part with the exception of guidance through issues of intervention. Here, we will devote a chapter to interventional radiology procedures from head to toe. Otherwise, we intend to provide a history-based guide to the neurological, pulmonary, cardiac, breast, gastrointestinal, genitourinary, and musculoskeletal organ systems. Unlike other books on this topic, we do not presume a known diagnosis but instead will offer guidance based on the clinical history, laboratory values, and physical findings as to the most efficacious imaging tests to make the correct diagnosis or evaluation of current therapy.

Philadelphia, PA, USA William R. Reinus, MD, MBA, FACR

Contents

Contributors

Surabhi Bajpai, DMRD Department of Radiology, Division of Abdominal Imaging and Intervention, Massachusetts General Hospital, Harvard Medical School, Boston, MA, USA

Robert Bronstein, MD Department of Radiology, Temple University Medical School, Philadelphia, PA, USA

Vineet Chib, MD Department of Radiology, Temple University Hospital, Philadelphia, PA, USA

Chandra A. Dass, MD Department of Radiology, Temple University Hospital, Philadelphia, PA, USA

Theresa Kaufman, DO Department of Radiology, Temple University Hospital, Philadelphia, PA, USA

Stephen E. Ling, MD Department of Radiology, Temple University Hospital, Philadelphia, PA, USA

Dillenia Reyes, MD Department of Radiology, Temple University Hospital, Philadelphia, PA, USA

Dushyant Sahani, MD Department of Radiology, Division of Abdominal Imaging and Intervention, Massachusetts General Hospital, Harvard Medical School, Boston, MA, USA

Pallav N. Shah, MD Division of Neuroradiology, Department of Radiology, Temple University Hospital, Philadelphia, PA, USA

Scott A. Simpson, MD Department of Radiology, Temple University Hospital, Philadelphia, PA, USA

Robert M. Steiner, MD Department of Radiology, Temple University Hospital, Philadelphia, PA, USA

Chapter 1
Imaging Modalities and Contrast Agents

Stephen E. Ling and Pallav N. Shah

Introduction

This chapter discusses the spectrum of available imaging studies employed in routine diagnostic imaging. Many of the associated advantages, deficiencies, concepts, and applications covered here can guide referring clinicians in selection of the appropriate imaging modality across organ systems, i.e., neurologic, cardiothoracic, gastrointestinal, genitourinary, vascular, and musculoskeletal (MSK). Regardless of the organ system, the choice of the appropriate study depends on multiple factors, including the clinical question to be addressed, the availability and accuracy of the imaging modality, study contraindications, risks of the imaging examination including those from contrast agent administration, and financial cost. Some very brief data regarding the Medicare reimbursements for several commonly ordered imaging examinations is also provided at the end of the chapter (Table 1.1).

It is important for clinicians to understand how contrast agents apply to imaging. Basic familiarity with common indications, significant contraindications and potential complications of contrast media use are essential for optimal patient care. We discuss the indications, contraindications, and risks of contrast agents that are routinely used in clinical practice today. This knowledge may be reinforced, and at times supplemented by radiologists in their role as consultants who are part of the medical team charged with quality diagnostic imaging management.

S.E. Ling, M.D. (✉)
Department of Radiology, Temple University Hospital, 3401 N. Broad Street, Philadelphia, PA 19140, USA
e-mail: Stephen.Ling@tuhs.temple.edu

P.N. Shah, M.D.
Division of Neuroradiology, Department of Radiology, Temple University Hospital, 3401 N. Broad Street, Philadelphia, PA 19140, USA
e-mail: pallav.shah@tuhs.temple.edu

W.R. Reinus (ed.), *Clinician's Guide to Diagnostic Imaging*,
DOI 10.1007/978-1-4614-8769-2_1, © Springer Science+Business Media New York 2014

Table 1.1 2012 Medicare reimbursement for various imaging modalities

Imaging modality	Reimbursement ($)[a]
CR	35
Skeletal survey	75
US limited (mass)	45
US complete (tendons, muscles, etc.)	130
CT (w/o, w/)	245–300
BS	275
BS (3 phase)	315
Labeled WBC study	375
MRI (w/o, w/ and w/o)	430–675
PET/CT	1,225

[a]2012 Medicare fee schedule: combined professional and technical fees (global fee)

Imaging Modalities

Overview

The most commonly used imaging technologies include conventional radiography (CR), computed tomography (CT), ultrasound (US), magnetic resonance imaging (MRI), and a variety of nuclear medicine studies (NM), each with a specific purpose (Table 1.2). While CR is typically a starting point for most evaluations in the chest, abdomen, and MSK system, this is not always the case. For example, soft tissue pathology generally is better evaluated by more advanced techniques, particularly MRI, US, and at times CT.

Conventional Radiography

Radiographs serve as the starting point in the imaging diagnosis of many categories of suspected pathology, e.g., pneumonia and congestive heart failure in the chest, small bowel obstruction and suspected free intraperitoneal air in the abdomen and especially for trauma, osteomyelitis, focal mass lesions, and arthropathies in the MSK system. Plain radiographs are inexpensive, widely available, and rapidly obtainable, even at the bedside if necessary. Disadvantages of radiographs include ionizing radiation and low contrast resolution making them unable to visualize most soft tissue abnormalities.

Ultrasound

US is less expensive than CT, MRI, and NM. In addition, it does not expose the patient to ionizing radiation, an important consideration particularly in children and

Table 1.2 Common diagnostic imaging modalities

Imaging modality	Advantages	Disadvantages and limitations
Conventional radiography (CR)	Very inexpensive Universally available Quickly obtained	Ionizing radiation Low contrast resolution Limited evaluation of soft tissues Projectional superimposition (2-D representation of 3-D anatomy and pathology)
Ultrasound (US)	Relative low cost (vs. CT, MRI, NM) No ionizing radiation Real time imaging Provocative patient maneuvers Guidance for numerous procedures	Operator-dependent Limited availability of well-trained, experienced MSK sonographers Narrow field of view Targeted, focused exam lacking the anatomic overview of other modalities
Computed tomography (CT)	Very wide availability Rapid image acquisition Largely "turnkey" and operator-independent Guidance for numerous procedures Excellent assessment of cortical bone (including erosion and destruction by tumor, infection, or inflammatory arthritis)	Ionizing radiation Potential adverse reactions if IV contrast needed Insensitive for bone marrow abnormalities
Magnetic resonance imaging (MRI)	No ionizing radiation Outstanding soft tissue contrast resolution Superb bone marrow evaluation	Expensive Comparative less availability Numerous contraindications Long imaging time, claustrophobia Nephrogenic systemic fibrosis (NSF) risk from gadolinium-based contrast agents (GBCAs) Relatively limited assessment of cortical bone (vs. CT)
Nuclear medicine (NM)	Less expensive than MRI	Ionizing radiation
Bone scintigraphy (BS)	Very large field of view (whole body assessment routinely performed)	Specificity limited (recently improved by adding CT)
Labeled leukocyte study (WBC)	Allows evaluation for multifocal disease Low resolution Sensitivity high Negative predictive value (NPV) high	Relatively limited in precise anatomic localization of pathology (better with SPECT, recent improvement with CT) Long study length (especially labeled WBC: imaging performed 2–4, 24, and possibly also 48 h postinjection)

(continued)

Table 1.2 (continued)

Imaging modality	Advantages	Disadvantages and limitations
Nuclear medicine (NM) FDG-PET	Very large field of view (whole body assessment routinely performed)	Ionizing radiation
	Allows evaluation for multifocal disease	Limited availability
	Sensitivity high	High cost
	Negative predictive value (NPV) high	Insurance reimbursement roadblocks
		Comparatively limited in precise anatomic localization of pathology (recently improved by addition of CT to create hybrid PET (PET/CT))

pregnant women. In appropriate well-trained, experienced hands, sonography excels in a number of applications. One of its main strengths is the ability to distinguish cystic from solid lesions. In addition, application of Doppler US enables visualization of a lesion's vascularity. US permits real time imaging, which allows for provocative maneuvers to detect pathology that is not well shown on static imaging studies. Examples of provocative maneuvers using dynamic real time US include compression of the gallbladder (sonographic Murphy sign) in evaluation of cholecystitis, elbow flexion to elicit ulnar nerve subluxation from the cubital tunnel, hip flexion to show snapping of the iliopsoas tendon in the groin, or compression of vessels to augment flow and show the absence of thrombus. US can also be used to guide interventional procedures including biopsy, e.g., liver or mass biopsy, and therapy such as injection of tendon sheaths, joints, bursae, and peritendinous soft tissues, e.g., the common extensor tendon origin at the lateral epicondyle of the elbow (tennis elbow).

US is operator-dependent. This means that specifically trained imagers are needed for this type of examination. US transducers have a narrow field of view, and so with today's scanning methods, it is possible to overlook pathology. Accordingly, US tends to be most successful when used to answer a specific clinical question with a focused examination of a limited anatomic region. Despite these limitations, the role of US continues to expand, especially the use of ultrasound-guided procedures.

Computed Tomography

CT technology has improved vastly since its introduction. It is now possible to image any part of the body with high spatial and moderate contrast resolution. Similar to CR, CT is readily and near universally available, even in rural locations, "after hours" and on weekends when other modalities are not available. As a result, CT has become the workhorse of diagnostic imaging. With newer scanners, it is possible to image large tissue volumes rapidly and if necessary repeatedly. This means that CT scans, either without or with the use of oral and/or intravenous contrast, can be configured to answer many clinical questions in every organ system. In fact, CT angiography has largely replaced conventional angiography for routine diagnosis.

When MRI is contraindicated or unavailable, CT often serves as a backup examination. In these cases, it is important to understand the differences in sensitivity and specificity between the two modalities for the clinical question being addressed. CT has better spatial resolution than MRI and is more sensitive at identifying calcium, but it has much lower contrast resolution compared with MRI, making its differentiation of structures poor in some parts of the body. These differences determine the value of attempting a CT as an alternative to MRI. This information will be covered further in the chapters on imaging of specific organ systems.

The main disadvantage of CT is its use of ionizing radiation. CT gives a higher dose of radiation to the patient than routine CR. Several studies have suggested that liberal use of CT will increase the incidence of neoplasms years on. In fact, today, dose levels with each scan are reported and recorded. So, while CT is an excellent diagnostic tool, the danger of high accumulated doses of radiation with this modality should temper its use. This is particularly true in the pediatric population where US should be employed whenever possible to avoid the radiation exposure from CT.

Magnetic Resonance Imaging

Although comparatively expensive, MRI is a commonly performed examination, particularly in neurologic, MSK, and to some extent cardiothoracic and abdominal disease. MRI has superior contrast resolution to other modalities and so is able to depict soft tissue structures that cannot be resolved by other imaging techniques.

As with CT, contrast agents are available for MR. These agents, primarily gadolinium-based, behave similarly to the iodinated contrast agents used for CT and fluoroscopic imaging. They have specific indications that will be discussed in each organ system chapter as appropriate. Other contrast agents are becoming available for specific use, for example, iron-based agents for the liver that are designed specifically for uptake by Kupffer cells. These are not yet widely available and have issues with toxicity.

MRI can accommodate a larger field of view than US, but it is important to understand that as the field of view increases, spatial resolution suffers. Spatial resolution is limited with MRI, and so the larger the field of view, the coarser the image detail obtained. In general, if a large area of the body needs to be imaged, or if there is suspicion for multifocal disease that requires imaging more than one anatomic location, nuclear imaging should be strongly considered in place of MRI. These scans, though often nonspecific, can include nearly the entire body in their field of view, something that is impractical with MRI. On the other hand, in some circumstances wide field of view MRI is useful, for example when surveying the skeleton for multiple myeloma.

Table 1.3 Study contrast media utilization[a] and contraindications in MRI/CT

Imaging modality	Indications (dosing route)	Contraindications (CI): absolute (A), relative (R)
MRI	Paraspinal, epidural abscess (IV)	Endocranial vascular clips (some) (A)
	Soft tissue abscess (IV)	Intra-aortic balloon pump (A)
	Intraosseous abscess (IV)	LVAD, RVAD (A)
	Bone sequestrum (IV)	Pulmonary artery catheter (A)
	Suspected early RA (IV)	Cardiac pacemaker (R)
	Synovitis, tenosynovitis (IV)	Implantable cardiovertor-defibrillator (R)
	Myositis (IV)	Capsule endoscopy device-Pillcam (A)
	Soft tissue mass (IV)	Hemostatic vascular clips (some) (A)
		Cochlear implants (R)
	Soft tissue necrosis, myonecrosis (IV)	Eye metallic foreign body (R)
	Osteonecrosis (IV)	Insulin pump (R)
	Direct MR arthrography (IArt)	GFR <15 mL/min (R)
	Indirect MR arthrography (IV)	ESRD on chronic dialysis (R)
	Vascular enhancement (IV)	GBCA use during pregnancy (R)
CT	Paraspinal, epidural abscess (IV)	Previous severe adverse reaction (e.g., profound vasovagal reaction, seizure, moderate and severe bronchospasm, laryngeal edema, severe hypotension, sudden cardiac arrest, cardiopulmonary complete collapse, and organ and system-specific adverse events)
	Soft tissue abscess (IV)	Acute kidney injury (AKI)
	Soft tissue mass (IV)	Oliguric dialysis patient (e.g., not ESRD anuric dialysis patient)
	Soft tissue necrosis, myonecrosis (IV)	
	CT arthrography (IAart)	
	Vascular enhancement (IV and IA)	

[a]Contrast agents: *MRI* gadolinium-based contrast agent (GBCA), *CT* iodinated contrast media; Administration: *IV* intravenous, *IA* intra-arterial, *IArt* intra-articular

There are a number of relative and absolute contraindications to the use of MRI. Because MRI uses strong magnetic fields, it can be dangerous to put patients with ferromagnetic devices and implants into a scanner (Table 1.3). First, depending on the device, its location in the body, and the duration that it's been implanted, the magnetic field may cause it to torque or dislodge. Second, depending on the configuration of the implanted device, the MR unit may cause it to generate microwaves and local tissue heating. Finally, the MR unit's magnetic field can trigger some pacemakers to go into test mode.

The list of contraindicated materials is a fluid one and a constant work in progress, with new additions (and removals) being made on a frequent basis. Many newer devices and implants are specifically designed to be MR compatible. Manufacturers usually provide patients with MR compatibility documentation to carry with them. Resources on the web, e.g., www.mrisafety.com maintain online up-to-date databases on the MR safety of medical devices. In order to use these, however, the patient must be able to provide relevant information regarding their device such as the manufacturer, model number, and date of manufacture. Finally, many radiologists experienced with MRI can help determine which types of devices are MR compatible.

Nuclear Medicine

NM studies had been designed to evaluate specific problems in every organ system whether the endocrine, e.g., thyroid scans, the MSK system, bone scans for osseous metastases or in the GI system, GI bleeding studies, and HIDA scans for gallbladder disease. Most nuclear medicine scans, though nonspecific, have the advantage of being comparatively sensitive and of providing physiologic information regarding target pathology. Furthermore, the recent addition of positron emission scanning (PET) alone and in combination with CT (PET/CT) has moved nuclear medicine into the fore of soft tissue tumor diagnosis and staging. This technique allows subtle areas of tumor to be discovered, diagnosed, staged, and so appropriately treated. PET/CT also has provided new tools for assessment of tissue viability, particularly in cardiac applications.

Contrast Media

Overview

Over the years, various types of contrast media have been used in attempts to improve the quality of imaging. These have provided significant additive value to the imaging modalities where they have been utilized. As a result, today contrast media are used on a routine, daily basis, especially iodinated contrast media for CT and radiography and gadolinium-based contrast agents (GBCAs) with MRI.

The majority of indications for use of intravenous (IV) contrast agents, regardless of whether it is iodinated contrast media or a GBCA, involve use of cross-sectional imaging for infectious, inflammatory, ischemic, and neoplastic pathology. For example, IV contrast material aids in the detection and delineation of fluid collections, regardless of their anatomic location. It also facilitates assessment of osseous and soft tissue viability, e.g., showing areas of necrosis in soft tissue and bone neoplasms and bony sequestra in chronic osteomyelitis. Inflammatory processes such as a variety of types of myositis, tenosynovitis, and synovitis are also typically better evaluated with IV contrast media. In addition, both iodinated and gadolinium (Gd)-based contrast agents very frequently enable determination of whether a soft tissue mass is cystic or solid in nature. The indications for utilization of IV contrast media are given in Table 1.3.

Contrast is also used intra-arterially (IA) for direct evaluation of the vessels. This is usually done with a catheter placed selectively into the vessel to be imaged. For unknown reasons, allergic contrast reactions to IA injected media are much less common than for IV injected contrast. Even so, because of the greater morbidity of direct contrast arteriography and the sophistication of current CT technology, IV contrast and CTA are more commonly used today.

Contrast media is commonly used intra-articularly as well, allowing the radiologist to actively distend the joint and thereby improve separation of intracapsular structures and enhance image resolution (Table 1.3). Intra-articular contrast injection is much more commonly performed with GBCA and MRI than iodinated contrast and CT, because of the inherent superiority of MRI in soft tissue contrast resolution. Regardless, as with IA injections, allergic reactions with intra-articular contrast are rare.

Contrast is also used intrathecally for myelography. Since the advent of MRI, the indications for myelogram have fallen markedly, but they are still performed in patients where there is a contraindication to MRI or there is adjacent metallic hardware that will induce obscuring MRI artifact.

Contrast agents are not without risk. Adverse side effects from the utilization of contrast media vary from relatively common, minor physiological disturbances that are almost always self-limited to rare, severe life-threatening anaphylactic reactions. In addition, iodinated contrast agents are nephrotoxic and are contraindicated in patients with renal failure as they may worsen renal function precipitously. GBCA are associated with nephrogenic systemic fibrosis (NSF) in patient with poor renal function. Therefore, prior to giving a patient contrast, their renal status should be assessed. Risks of a reaction should be considered when making decisions regarding patient management [1].

Preceding the actual imaging of a patient, the radiologist in conjunction with the ordering physician should address a few preliminary considerations for any given patient. Specifically, the radiologist in particular should make best efforts to determine if there is an appropriate indication for the requested study, identify relative contraindications and pertinent risk factors that may increase the likelihood of an adverse reaction to contrast administration, and possess sufficient knowledge of alternative imaging modalities [1].

Risk Factors Associated with Iodinated Contrast Media

Risk factors for adverse reactions to IV iodinated contrast material include prior reaction, known allergy (history of prior allergic-type reaction particularly if moderate to severe in degree), asthma, renal insufficiency, and cardiovascular disease (if the patient has congestive heart failure symptoms or angina, severe aortic stenosis, severe cardiomyopathy, or primary pulmonary hypertension) [1]. There are a number of miscellaneous risk factors. One of these is multiple myeloma, which is known to cause irreversible renal failure from renal tubular protein precipitation and aggregation when high-osmolality contrast media (HOCM) is used in these patients. Other potential miscellaneous risk factors include β-adrenergic blockers, which are associated with more frequent and more severe adverse events, and pheochromocytoma, where an increase in serum catecholamine levels may be seen after IV injection of HOCM resulting in a hypertensive crisis [1].

Premedication

Patients who are known to be at higher risk for an acute allergic-type contrast reaction and for whom a scan is needed should be considered for premedication prior to a scan. Many adverse reactions are associated with direct release of histamine and other mediators from circulating basophils and eosinophils [1]. Studies have shown that IV steroids suppress whole blood histamine and show a reduction in circulating basophils and eosinophils [2].

This observation provides a scientific basis for the use of IV steroids in "at risk" patients during emergency situations. Corticosteroids have been shown to have a prophylactic effect for adverse reactions to contrast media in certain circumstances. Some corticosteroid preventative effect may be obtained as soon as 1 h after IV injection of corticosteroids, but experimental data support a much better prophylactic effect if the examination is not performed until at least 4–6 h after giving premedication [3–5]. No clinical studies have demonstrated unequivocally prevention of contrast reactions using short-term IV corticosteroid premedication. If the time frame available for utilizing corticosteroids is too short and the risks of a major reaction judged to be small, some physicians will forgo them and administer only an antihistamine before contrast use [4].

Whether in the emergent or elective setting, it is most important to target premedication to those who, in the past, have had moderately severe or severe reactions that required treatment. Unfortunately, studies thus far have shown that the majority of patients who benefit from premedication are those who have had minor contrast reactions that typically require no or minimal medical intervention [5]. To date, randomized controlled clinical trials have not demonstrated premedication protection against severe life-threatening adverse reactions [3, 6, 7].

Oral administration of steroids is preferable to IV administration, and prednisone and methylprednisolone are equally effective. Regardless of the route of corticosteroid administration, ideally the steroids should be given at least 6 h prior to the injection of contrast media. It is unclear if steroid administration within 3 h of contrast media administration reduces adverse reactions. Some recommended and commonly used dosing schedules for premedication in either the elective or

Elective Premedication

Two frequently used regiments are:

1. Prednisone – 50 mg by mouth at 13 hours, 7 hours, and 1 hour before contrast media injection, plus

   Diphenhydramine (Benadryl®) – 50 mg intravenously, intramuscularly, or by mouth 1 hour before contrast medium.

or

2. Methylprednisolone (Medrol®) – 32 mg by mouth 12 hours and 2 hours before contrast media injection. An anti-histamine (as in option 1) can also be added to this regimen injection.

   If the patient is unable to take oral medication, 200 mg of hydrocortisone intravenously may be substituted for oral prednisone in the Greenberger protocol.

Emergency Premedication (In Decreasing Order of Desirability)

1. Methylprednislone sodium succinate (Solu-Medrol®) 40 mg or hydrocortisone sodium succinate (Solu-Cortef®) 200 mg intravenously every 4 hours (q4h) until contrast study required plus diphenhydramine 50 mg IV 1 hour prior to contrast injection.

2. Dexamethasone sodium sulfate (Decadron®) 7.5 mg or betamethasone 6.0 mg intravenously q4h until contrast study must be done in patent with known allergy to methylpred-nisolone, aspirin, or non-steroidal anti-inflammatory drugs, especially if asthmatic. Also diphenhydramine 50 mg IV 1 hour prior to contrast injection.

3. Omit steroids entirely and give diphenhydramine 50 mg IV.

   Note: IV steroids have not been shown to be effective when administered less than 4 to 6 hours prior to contrast injection.

Fig. 1.1 Recommended premedication regimens to reduce frequency and/or severity of reactions to iodinated contrast media (From: [1] Manual on Contrast Media, Version 8. Reston, VA: American College of Radiology; 2012)

emergent setting are included below (Fig. 1.1) [1]. Further, oral or intravenous administration of an H-1 antihistamine, e.g., diphenhydramine, either alone or as a supplement to corticosteroids may reduce the frequency of urticaria, angioedema, and respiratory symptoms [1].

Breakthrough Reactions

Repeat contrast reactions in premedicated patients are termed breakthrough reactions. Breakthrough reactions most often are similar to the index reaction. Patients with a previous mild contrast reaction have an extremely low risk of developing a severe breakthrough reaction. The majority of low-osmolality contrast material

(LOCM) injections in premedicated patients who had prior breakthrough reactions will not result in a repeat breakthrough reaction [8, 9]. On the other hand, although there is a decrease in the overall adverse events after steroid premedication prior to contrast injection, studies have shown no decrease in the incidence of repeat severe adverse events [10].

Adverse Events Following Iodinated Contrast Media Administration

The frequency of adverse events after administration of iodinated contrast media can be decreased by utilization of nonionic LOCM [11–13]. Several studies have reported overall adverse reaction rates or allergic-like reaction rates ranging from 0.18 to 0.7 % [1]. HOCM use historically has been associated with a much higher rate of acute adverse reactions of 5–15 % [1], but HOCM is not used commonly anymore.

Acute adverse events after iodinated contrast media use can be subdivided into several categories, allergic-like or physiologic, and these are classified further as mild, moderate, or severe (Fig. 1.2) [1]. Other reactions are organ or system-specific reactions (Fig. 1.3) [1].

Allergic-like reactions are clinically identical to an anaphylactic reaction to any other drug or allergen [12–14]. Physiologic reactions include commonly occurring but usually mild and self-limited vasovagal reactions like hypotension with bradycardia [13], as well as rare cardiovascular events such as arrhythmias, impaired myocardial contractility [13–15], and both cardiogenic and noncardiogenic pulmonary edema [16].

Mild adverse reactions are frequently nonallergic-like physiologic responses (e.g., nausea, vomiting, and a feeling of warmth). Whether allergic-like or nonallergic-like, these mild effects usually do not require medical treatment, but they do have the potential to evolve into a more severe reaction and so must be monitored [1]. Moderate adverse events may also be allergic-like, e.g., severe urticaria/erythema, bronchospasm, moderate tongue/facial swelling, transient hypotension with tachycardia, or nonallergic-like, e.g., significant vasovagal reaction. In most instances, these adverse reactions are not immediately life-threatening. Nonetheless, they often require medical treatment. As with mild adverse reactions, events in the moderate group have the potential to worsen, in the latter case resulting in significant morbidity or even mortality [1]. Severe adverse events are usually allergic-like, but also may be physiologic. Acute adverse advents that fall under the category of serious reactions occur in only 0.01–0.02 % of imaging studies where LOCM is used [17]. Although these allergic reactions are quite rare, they may be life-threatening, and the majority of patients require treatment. Severe reactions include altered mental status, respiratory distress due to severe bronchospasm or laryngeal edema, severe hypotension, and sudden cardiac arrest. Complete

Categories of Reactions

Classification of Severity and Manifestations of Adverse Reactions to Contrast Media

Mild

Signs and symptoms appear self-limited without evidence of progression (e.g., limited urticaria with mild pruritis, transient nausea, one episode of emesis) and include:

- Nausea, vomiting
- Cough
- Warmth
- Headache
- Dizziness
- Shaking
- Altered taste
- Itching
- Pallor
- Flushing
- Chills
- Sweats
- Rash, hives
- Nasal stuffiness
- Swelling: eyes, face
- Anxiety

Treatment: Requires observation to confirm resolution and/or lack of progression but usually no treatment. Patient reassurance is usually helpful.

Moderate

Signs and symptoms are more pronounced. Moderate degree of clinically evident focal or systemic signs or symptoms, including:

- Tachycardia/bradycardia
- Hypertension
- Generalized or diffues erythema
- Dyspnea
- Bronchospasm, wheezing
- Laryngeal edema
- Mild hypotension

Treatment: Clinical findings in moderate reactions frequently require prompt treatment. These situtaions require close, careful observation for possible progression to a life-threatening event.

Severe

Signs and symptoms are often life-threatening, including:

- Laryngeal edema (severe or rapdidly progressing)
- Profound hypotension
- Clinically manifest arrhythmias
- Convulsions
- Unresponsiveness
- Cardiopulmonary arrest

Treatment: Requires prompt recognition and aggressive treatment, manifestations and treatment frequently require hospitalization.

Note: The above classifications (mild, moderate, severe) do not attempts to distiguish between allergic-like and non-allergic like reactions. Rather, they encompass the specrum of adverse events that can be seen following the intravascular injection of contast media.

Fig. 1.2 Categories of reactions to contrast media administration (From: [1] Manual on Contrast Media, Version 8. Reston, VA: American College of Radiology; 2012)

cardiopulmonary collapse is extremely rare. Less frequent than their allergic-like counterparts, severe nonallergic-like adverse events are also possible and usually necessitate medical management other than epinephrine. These include prominent vasovagal reactions, pulmonary edema, and seizures [1].

Organ and System-Specific Adverse Effects from the Administration of Iodine-Based or Gadolinium-Based Contrast Agents

Individual organs can manifest isolated adverse effects caused by the administration of contrast media.

Adrenal Glands
- Hypertension (in patients with pheochromocytoma after intra-arterial injection)

Brain
- Headache
- Confusion
- Dizziness
- Seizure
- Rigors
- Lost or diminished consciousness
- Lost or diminished vision

Gastrointestinal Tract
- Nausea
- Vomiting
- Diarrhea
- Intestinal cramping

Heart
- Hypotension
- Dysrhythmia (asystole, ventricular fibrillation/ventricular tachycardia)
- Pulseless electrical activity (PEA)
- Acute congestive heart failure

Kidney
- Oliguria
- Hypertension
- Contrast-induced nephropathy (CIN)

Pancreas
- Swelling / pancreatitis

Respiratory System
- Laryngeal edema
- Bronchospasm
- Pulmonary edema

Salivary Glands
- Swelling / parotitis

Skin and Soft Tissues
- Pain
- Edema
- Flushing
- Erythema
- Urticaria
- Pruritus
- Compartment syndrome (from extravasation)
- Nephrogenic Systemic Fibrosis (NSF)

Thyroid
- Exacerbation of thyrotoxicosis

Vascular System
- Hemorrhage (due to direct vascular trauma from contrast injection or from the reduction in clotting ability
- Thrombophlebitis

Fig. 1.3 Organ and system-specific adverse events after administration of iodine-based or gadolinium-based contrast media (From: [1] Manual on Contrast Media, Version 8. Reston, VA: American College of Radiology; 2012)

Organ and system-specific adverse reactions refer to adverse effects on a more isolated basis. Neurologic, cardiovascular, and renal abnormalities account for the majority of the adverse events in this group. Contrast-induced nephrotoxicity (CIN) is the most significant organ-specific adverse effect and is discussed in more detail below [1].

Risk factors for acute adverse events following contrast administration can be identified for allergic-like reactions. Prior allergic-like reaction is the biggest risk factor [11, 12], with a reported incidence of recurrent adverse event as high as 35 % [18]. Patients with asthma or a history of atopia also are at increased risk for adverse reaction, although the risk is not as high as in those with history of prior allergic-like event [13–15].

Non-Acute, Delayed Adverse Reactions

Nearly all life-threatening iodinated contrast media reactions occur immediately or within the first 20 min after contrast media injection [1]. Notwithstanding, non-acute adverse reactions to iodinated contrast media may arise between 3 h and 2 days, but have been seen as early as 30 min or as late as 7 days after contrast administration [18, 19]. These delayed adverse events may be allergic-like or nonallergic-like, but they are most commonly allergic-like and cutaneous in nature, presenting as urticaria and/or a persistent rash. The incidence of these events is not rare with reports ranging from 0.5 to 14 % [19, 20]. Most cases are self-limited and require minimal if any treatment other than symptomatic support [1]. Severe delayed adverse events are extraordinarily rare but may occur. The recurrence rate of delayed contrast reactions upon reexposure to contrast material is not known, but anecdotally may be higher than 25 % [21]. It is not clear if corticosteroid premedication is indicated before a subsequent contrast-enhanced study in patients with a history of delayed allergic-like contrast reaction [1].

Contrast-Induced Nephrotoxicity

CIN is a sudden deterioration in renal function after recent intravascular administration of iodinated contrast medium in the absence of another nephrotoxic event [22]. CIN is either exceedingly rare or does not occur with use of GBCAs [1]. The pathophysiology of CIN and associated acute kidney injury is not well understood. Fortunately, CIN usually follows a course of transient asymptomatic elevation in serum creatinine, beginning to rise within 1 day, peaking within 4 days, and typically returning to baseline within 7–10 days. Chronic renal dysfunction is unusual unless other risk factors are present [1].

The most unequivocal, clear risk of developing CIN is preexisting renal insufficiency [23]. Numerous other proposed risk factors, including diabetes mellitus, hypertension, and multiple doses of iodinated contrast over a short time period (e.g., <24 h), have not been convincingly confirmed in the literature. Numerous papers have found the incidence of CIN is less with IV than IA iodinated contrast media.

At the present time, the practice guideline of the American College of Radiology (ACR) for the use of IV iodinated contrast material with regard to the potential risk of CIN is that there is insufficient data to set a specific recommended threshold level for serum creatinine above which iodinated contrast should not be given. Most institutions withhold contrast when the creatinine is greater than or equal to 2.0 mg/dL [1]. Many use lower levels as the cut off.

Patients older than age 60, those with hypertension, diabetes mellitus, and known renal risk factors, including a history of a single kidney, renal transplant, kidney surgery, renal cancer, and dialysis, should be routinely screened with a serum creatinine level before receiving iodinated contrast [24, 25]. Use of less nephrotoxic

LOCM [26] and adequate patient hydration prior to the study [27] are standard practices in an attempt to limit the possibility of CIN. Several pharmacological agents, including IV sodium bicarbonate, *N*-acetylcysteine, diuretics, theophylline, and fenoldopam, thus far have been unconvincing as far as their efficacy with regard to preventing CIN [1].

Metformin

The anti-hyperglycemic agent, Metformin, has been associated with a rare but life-threatening complication in patients who receive intravascular iodinated contrast. The kidneys eliminate this anti-hyperglycemic agent, excreting approximately 90 % of a dose within the first 24 h. Instances have been reported in which patients taking metformin develop lactic acidosis after receiving iodinated contrast media [1]. The apparent cause is that contrast-induced decline in renal function leads to elevated Metformin levels which in turn cause increased production of lactic acid by the GI tract. Although this complication is estimated to occur at a rate of no more than 0.1 cases per 1,000 patient years, when Metformin-associated lactic acidosis occurs, mortality is approximately 50 % [1].

In almost all reported cases of this serious adverse reaction, lactic acidosis likely developed because associated other contraindications and comorbidities for the drug were overlooked, i.e., renal or cardiovascular disease, but also decreased lactate metabolism states from hepatic dysfunction and alcohol abuse, as well as increased anaerobic metabolism resulting from sepsis or severe infection. In properly selected patients, there have been no documented cases of Metformin-associated lactic acidosis [1].

The ACR recommends that patients taking Metformin who are scheduled to receive iodinated contrast media be stratified into three groups. This stratification of patients should be done on the basis of pre-examination renal function, and known comorbidities associated with decreased lactate metabolism or increased anaerobic metabolism. Management of the individual patient will vary depending on their classification category, including possible Metformin discontinuation, continued assessment of renal function following the imaging study, and the timing of the reinstitution of Metformin [1].

Adverse Events After Gadolinium-Based Contrast Agent Administration

The incidence of acute adverse events after administration of a routine IV dose gadolinium chelate ranges from 0.07 to 2.4 %. The vast majority of these reactions is mild and resembles adverse reactions from use of iodinated contrast media. Severe, life-threatening allergic or nonallergic anaphylactic reactions are extremely rare with an incidence of 0.001–0.01 %. Fatal reactions to gadolinium chelate agents, although possible, are exceedingly rare [1].

As with iodinated contrast media, a history of prior adverse reaction to GBCA places the patient at much greater risk (approximately 8×) for a repeat adverse advent. Similarly, patients with asthma and other allergies have an increased incidence of allergic-like adverse events with GBCA, as high as 3.7 % [1].

When used at approved dosages, there is no significant evidence to suggest that GBCA is nephrotoxic. Instead, use of a GBCA in patients with advanced renal dysfunction (those with ESRD and a creatinine clearance of <15 cm^3/min, but also others with a creatanine clearance of 15–30 cm^3/min) places the patient at significant risk for the development of NSF. GBCA crosses the blood-placenta barrier into the fetal blood stream, and it may accumulate in amniotic fluid, thus making its use in pregnant patients a relative contraindication [1].

Nephrogenic Systemic Fibrosis

The first cases of NSF were diagnosed in 1997, and the first published report of 14 cases appeared back in 2000 [28]. Despite this, NSF only recently has received considerable attention in the medical community, largely because of identification of a possible link with GBCA agents that have been widely used in MRI for the past 20 years. In 2006, several groups made the observation of a strong association between GBCA administration and development of NSF in patients with advanced renal disease, and it is now widely accepted that exposure to GBCA is a prerequisite to develop NSF.

The disorder was initially termed nephrogenic fibrosing dermopathy given the prominence of its skin manifestations, which include thick, hard skin starting in the extremities, sometimes extending to the torso, and resembling that of progressive systemic sclerosis [29]. After multiple autopsy case reports on patients with the disease that described myocardial, pericardial, and pleural fibrosis, along with nerve and skeletal muscle involvement, nephrogenic fibrosing dermopathy was renamed NSF to emphasize the non-dermatological features of the disorder [30]. Patients afflicted by NSF not only have wooden, unpinchable skin; they also may have scleral plaques, joint contractures, muscle weakness, pruritus, and sharp pain. Arriving at a confident diagnosis of NSF in a given individual is a complex undertaking that relies on the expertise of specialist physicians, clinical history and physical examination, and tissue sampling. More specifically, the diagnosis of NSF involves physical exam of the patient by a seasoned dermatologist or rheumatologist, and histopathologic assessment of skin biopsy tissue by an experienced dermatopathologist [31, 32].

The incidence of NSF in much of the literature varies from 3 to 7 % in patients receiving Omniscan (gadodiamide) [31], the GBCA administered in a very large percentage of reported NSF cases. One study reported an incidence of NSF of 18 % for patients in the highest risk group (GFR <15 mL/min) [33]. About 5 % of patients with NSF are afflicted by the fulminant subtype of the disorder. These patients experience rapid progression of disease including accelerated loss of mobility and severe pain [32]. In those cases where NSF is fatal, visceral involvement is the most common cause of death, especially cardiovascular events [34].

In 2008, Knopp et al. observed that all documented cases of NSF to date had acute or chronic renal insufficiency (GFR <30 mL/min); were related to acute renal insufficiency in hepatorenal syndrome; or arose perioperatively in liver transplantation patients [31]. Most cases of biopsy-proven NSF reported in the peer-reviewed literature are associated with ESRD (GFR <15 mL/min) (85 %), Omniscan (gadodiamide) GBCA, exposure to a single high dose, or more commonly multiple doses of contrast, within a 6 month time frame, the last exposure to contrast within 6 months, and current or previous dialysis (62 %) [31]. A high total cumulative lifetime dose of GBCA increases the risk of NSF. There has been only one published case report of a patient with GFR >30 mL/min acquiring NSF [35] (Table 1.4).

Cases of NSF can be categorized as confounded or unconfounded. Confounded cases are those in which the patient has a history of having received more than one type of GBCA prior to onset of NSF, while in unconfounded cases the patient was exposed to only a single GBCA. In a meta-analysis of the literature published in 2008, out of 168 unconfounded cases of NSF, the overwhelming majority involved Omniscan (gadodiamide) (93 %), distantly followed by Magnevist (gadopentetate dimeglumine) (5 %) and then Optimark (gadoversetamide) (2 %) [36]. Other brands of GBCAs have been associated with few, if any, confirmed cases of NSF (Fig. 1.4) [1]. Thus, the precise relationship between NSF and different formulations of GBCAs is controversial and incompletely understood.

Since most patients, including those with ESRD, do not develop NSF, other possible triggers, cotriggers, or predisposing conditions have been suggested, such as vascular surgery, hypercoagulability or thrombotic events, high-dose erythropoietin administration, immunosuppression, infection, proinflammatory state, metabolic acidosis, and elevated serum levels of iron, calcium, and phosphorus [1, 31, 32] (Table 1.4). To date, there is no clear evidence that any of these factors play a role in the development of NSF.

It is now widely accepted that GBCA exposure is a prerequisite for the development of NSF [1]. The exact mechanism by which GBCA exerts its effect in NSF is unknown, or at least not well understood. The most favored theory is that the gadolinium (Gd) ion dissociates from its chelate and then binds other anions such as phosphate producing an insoluble precipitate that remains in the skin and other tissues for weeks, months, or even years [1, 32], thus inciting a fibrotic reaction.

Since the medical community does not know why only a minority of patients at risk develop NSF, caution should be exercised when administering GBCA in patients with advanced renal failure. Assessment of the risks and benefits of GBCA administration should be performed for each patient via close consultation between radiologist and clinician and GBCA administered only to patients where the information provided by its use is both essential to patient care and unable to be obtained by other means [31]. If a decision is made to utilize GBCA, the imaging study should be monitored by the radiologist. If the initial non-contrast images

Table 1.4 Nephrogenic systemic fibrosis (NSF)

Signs and symptoms	Epidemiology	Pathophysiology	Triggers, cotriggers, and predisposing conditions	Notes
Thick, hard, wooden skin	ESRD (GFR <15 mL/min): 85 % of patients with NSF	Exact mechanism of NSF development unknown or poorly understood	Vascular surgery	Close consultation between radiologist and clinician essential to appropriate risk-benefit assessment
Pruritus	Symptom onset within days to 6 months of last exposure	Most widely favored theory:	Hypercoagulability	Perform contrast study only if the desired information is essential and cannot be obtained by other means
Lungs, heart, esophagus, and skeletal muscles Myocardial, pericardial, and pleural fibrosis	Exposure to single high dose or multiple doses within 6 month time frame	Gadolinium (Gd) ion dissociates from its chelate, free Gd binds other anions, and resultant insoluble precipitate deposits in soft tissues	High dose erythropoietin	Radiologist should monitor study and determine if non-contrast images are diagnostically adequate (obviating need for GBCA)
Joint contracture	High total cumulative lifetime dose of GBCA increases risk	GBCA able to cross the blood-placenta barrier into the fetus, and likely accumulates in amniotic fluid (relative contraindication)	Immunosuppression	Coordinate for hemodialysis (~2 and possibly 24 h after MRI) to enhance GBCA elimination
Muscle weakness Death (usually due to visceral involvement)	Dialysis: current or past NSF incidence: ~3–7 % Rapidly progressive NSF: <5 % Most common agent used in unconfounded cases of NSF: Omniscan		Infection Metabolic acidosis High Fe, Ca^{2+}, P levels	

Group I: Agents associated with the greatest number of NSF cases:
Gadodiamide (Omniscan® – GE Healthcare)
Gadopentetate dimeglumine (Magnevist® – Bayer HealthCare Pharmaceuticals)
Gadoversetamide (OptiMARK®–Covidien)
Group II: Agents associated with few, if any, unconfounded cases of NSF:
Gadobenate dimeglumine (MultiHance® – Bracco Diagnostics)
Gadoteridol (ProHance® – Bracco Diagnostics)
Gadoteric acid (Dotarem® – Guerbet – as of this writing not FDA-approved for use in the U.S.)
Gadobutrol (Gadavist® – Bayer HealthCare Pharmaceuticals)
Group III: Agents which have only recently appeared on the market in th US:
Gadofosvest (Ablavar® – Lantheus Medical Imaging)
Gadoxetic acid (Eovist® – Bayer HealthCare Pharmaceuticals)

There is limited data for Group III agents, although, to date, few, if any, unconfounded cases of NSF have been reported.

Fig. 1.4 Association between various Gadolinium-based contrast agent (GBCA) and cases of NSF (From: [1] Manual on Contrast Media, Version 8. Reston, VA: American College of Radiology; 2012)

are diagnostically adequate, the radiologist can cancel the planned utilization of Gd contrast [31].

The radiologist and clinician can also coordinate post-MRI hemodialysis for patients following a study in which GBCA is administered. Dialysis should be performed approximately 2 h and if possible again at 24 h after the MRI to accelerate GBCA elimination. It should be noted, however, that there are currently no data showing that reducing free Gd levels with dialysis decreases the risk of developing NSF [31].

Administration of Iodinated Contrast Media and GBCA in Pregnancy

Studies in the medical literature focusing on fetal effects of iodinated contrast media (both ionic and nonionic) and GBCAs during pregnancy are limited. Potential negative effects on the human embryo and fetus are incompletely understood. Both iodinated contrast agents and gadolinium-based MR contrast media, when administered in doses typically used in clinical practice, cross the human placenta and enter the fetus in measurable quantities [37, 38].

After entering the fetal blood stream, contrast agents are excreted via the urine into the amniotic fluid. This is then swallowed by the fetus [39], a small percentage is absorbed by the GI tact, and the rest returned back to the amniotic fluid. The cycle is then repeated innumerable times. Currently, it is not known how quickly contrast media is cleared from the amniotic fluid.

In-vivo tests in animals have shown no evidence of either mutagenic or teratogenic effects with iodinated low-osmolality contrast media (LOCM). No adequate and well-controlled studies of the teratogenic effects of iodinated contrast agents in pregnant women have been performed. At the current time, there is insufficient evidence to conclude whether or not iodinated contrast media pose a risk to the fetus. Policies and procedures designed to identify pregnant patients prior to exposure to ionizing radiation (e.g., CT) also should be used to assess the medical necessity for administration of iodinated contrast media in these patients.

No well-controlled studies of the teratogenic effects of GBCA in pregnant women have been performed. This class of contrast agent poses more difficulties than iodinated contrast media, largely because less is known about potential fetal toxicities. Gadolinium chelates may accumulate in the amniotic fluid and remain for an indefinite period of time. It is also possible that toxic-free gadolinium can dissociate from its chelate in this environment. Potential toxic effects from exposure to free Gd ions are unknown, as is association between free gadolinium ions and development of NSF in the fetus.

As a result, GBCA should not be used routinely in pregnant patients. The same precautions with the use of GBCA in ESRD patients should be exercised in pregnant women as well. The radiologist should confer with the clinician to be sure that the following criteria are met: (1) the diagnostic information expected to be provided by the MRI cannot be acquired without the use of IV contrast media or by using other imaging modalities, (2) the information needed affects the care of the patient and fetus during the pregnancy, and (3) the referring physician feels that it is not prudent to wait until after parturition to obtain this information.

Administration of Iodinated Contrast Media and GBCA to Breast-Feeding Mothers

Often, patients and/or their physicians have concerns about potential toxicity to the infant caused by contrast media that is excreted into the mother's breast milk. Mothers who are breast-feeding should be given the opportunity to make an informed decision as to whether to continue or temporarily abstain from breast-feeding after receiving intravascularly administered iodinated contrast media or GBCA. The literature on the excretion of iodinated contrast agents (both ionic and nonionic) and GBCA into breast milk and the subsequent gastrointestinal absorption of these agents from breast milk is limited, but sufficient for the ACR to construct a position statement on this topic.

A number of studies have reported that less than 1 % of the maternal dose of iodinated contrast material is excreted into breast milk during the first 24 h. Furthermore, less than 1 % of the contrast medium in the breast milk that the infant ingests is absorbed by its gastrointestinal tract [40–42]. Therefore, the expected dose of contrast media absorbed by an infant from ingested breast milk is less than

0.01 % of the intravascular dose administered to the mother. This amount of contrast material represents less than 1 % of the recommended contrast dose for an infant undergoing an imaging study.

The literature reports that only 0.04 % of the maternal GBCA dose is excreted into the breast milk in the first 24 h. As with iodinated contrast material, less than 1 % of the GBCA in breast milk ingested by the infant is absorbed by its gastrointestinal tract [43, 44]. Thus, the expected dose of GBCA absorbed from ingested breast milk by an infant is less than 0.0004 % of the dose received by the child's mother. This amount of GBCA is 0.04 % of the permitted adult or pediatric (2 years or older) IV dose.

Although free gadolinium is neurotoxic, it is safe for use in most adults and children when complexed to one of a variety of chelates. However, because it is not known how much, if any, of the gadolinium in breast milk is in unchelated form, the infant may be at risk due to direct toxicity from free Gd. Potential risk also includes allergic sensitization or reaction. So far, these are mainly theoretical type concerns.

Because of the very low percentage of iodinated contrast agent or GBCA that is excreted into the breast milk and absorbed by the infant's GI tract, and absence of evidence in the literature that ingestion of this amount of contrast has toxic effects, the ACR position on this issue is that it is safe for the mother and infant to continue breast-feeding after receiving a contrast agent. If the mother remains concerned about contrast media administration having potential ill effects on her infant, a reasonable option is to temporarily abstain from breast-feeding after receiving contrast. Both iodinated contrast agents and gadolinium contrast media have a plasma half-life of approximately 2 h, which results in clearance of nearly 100 % of contrast media from the bloodstream within 24 h. As a result, the mother can discontinue breast-feeding for 24 h, but she must actively express and discard her breast milk during that period.

References

1. Manual on Contrast Media, Version 8. Reston, VA: American College of Radiology; 2012.
2. Dunsky EH, Zweiman B, Fischler E, Levy DA. Early effects of corticosteroids on basophils, leukocyte histamine, and tissue histamine. J Allergy Clin Immunol. 1979;63:426–32.
3. Morcos SK. Review article: Acute serious and fatal reactions to contrast media: our current understanding. Br J Radiol. 2005;78:686–93.
4. Lasser EC. Pretreatment with corticosteroids to prevent reactions to i.v. contrast material: overview and implications. AJR Am J Roentgenol. 1988;150:257–9.
5. Lasser EC, Berry CC, Mishkin MM, Williamson B, Zheutlin N, Silverman JM. Pretreatment with corticosteroids to prevent adverse reactions to nonionic contrast media. AJR Am J Roentgenol. 1994;162:523–6.
6. Brockow K, Christiansen C, Kanny G, et al. Management of hypersensitivity reactions to iodinated contrast media. Allergy. 2005;60:150–8.
7. Tramer MR, von Elm E, Loubeyre P, Hauser C. Pharmacological prevention of serious anaphylactic reactions due to iodinated contrast media: systematic review. Bmj. 2006;333:675.
8. Davenport MS, Cohan RH, Caoili EM, Ellis JH. Repeat contrast medium reactions in premedicated patients: frequency and severity. Radiology. 2009;253:372–9.

9. Freed KS, Leder RA, Alexander C, DeLong DM, Kliewer MA. Breakthrough adverse reactions to low-osmolar contrast media after steroid premedication. AJR Am J Roentgenol. 2001;176: 1389–92.
10. Greenberger PA, Patterson R. The prevention of immediate generalized reactions to radiocontrast media in high-risk patients. J Allergy Clin Immunol. 1991;87:867–72.
11. Bettmann MA, Heeren T, Greenfield A, Goudey C. Adverse events with radiographic contrast agents: results of the SCVIR Contrast Agent Registry. Radiology. 1997;203:611–20.
12. Brockow K. Contrast media hypersensitivity–scope of the problem. Toxicology. 2005;209: 189–92.
13. Bush WH, Swanson DP. Acute reactions to intravascular contrast media: types, risk factors, recognition, and specific treatment. AJR Am J Roentgenol. 1991;157:1153–61.
14. Cohan RH, Dunnick NR. Intravascular contrast media: adverse reactions. AJR Am J Roentgenol. 1987;149:665–70.
15. Lieberman PL, Seigle RL. Reactions to radiocontrast material. Anaphylactoid events in radiology. Clin Rev Allergy Immunol. 1999;17:469–96.
16. Bouachour G, Varache N, Szapiro N, L'Hoste P, Harry P, Alquier P. Noncardiogenic pulmonary edema resulting from intravascular administration of contrast material. AJR Am J Roentgenol. 1991;157:255–6.
17. Katayama H, Yamaguchi K, Kozuka T, Takashima T, Seez P, Matsuura K. Adverse reactions to ionic and nonionic contrast media. A report from the Japanese Committee on the Safety of Contrast Media. Radiology. 1990;175:621–8.
18. Meth MJ, Maibach HI. Current understanding of contrast media reactions and implications for clinical management. Drug Saf. 2006;29:133–41.
19. Christiansen C, Pichler WJ, Skotland T. Delayed allergy-like reactions to X-ray contrast media: mechanistic considerations. Eur Radiol. 2000;10:1965–75.
20. Loh S, Bagheri S, Katzberg RW, Fung MA, Li CS. Delayed adverse reaction to contrast-enhanced CT: a prospective single-center study comparison to control group without enhancement. Radiology. 2010;255:764–71.
21. Webb JA, Stacul F, Thomsen HS, Morcos SK. Late adverse reactions to intravascular iodinated contrast media. Eur Radiol. 2003;13:181–4.
22. Katzberg RW, Newhouse JH. Intravenous contrast medium-induced nephrotoxicity: is the medical risk really as great as we have come to believe? Radiology. 2010;256:21–8.
23. Abujudeh HH, Gee MS, Kaewlai R. In emergency situations, should serum creatinine be checked in all patients before performing second contrast CT examinations within 24 hours? J Am Coll Radiol. 2009;6:268–73.
24. Choyke PL, Cady J, DePollar SL, Austin H. Determination of serum creatinine prior to iodinated contrast media: is it necessary in all patients? Tech Urol. 1998;4:65–9.
25. Tippins RB, Torres WE, Baumgartner BR, Baumgarten DA. Are screening serum creatinine levels necessary prior to outpatient CT examinations? Radiology. 2000;216:481–4.
26. Barrett BJ, Carlisle EJ. Metaanalysis of the relative nephrotoxicity of high- and low-osmolality iodinated contrast media. Radiology. 1993;188:171–8.
27. Solomon RJ, Natarajan MK, Doucet S, et al. Cardiac Angiography in Renally Impaired Patients (CARE) study: a randomized double-blind trial of contrast-induced nephropathy in patients with chronic kidney disease. Circulation. 2007;115:3189–96.
28. Cowper SE, Robin HS, Steinberg SM, Su LD, Gupta S, LeBoit PE. Scleromyxoedema-like cutaneous disease in renal-dialysis patients. Lancet. 2000;356:1000–1.
29. Mendoza FA, Artlett CM, Sandorfi N, Latinis K, Piera-Velazquez S, Jimenez SA. Description of 12 cases of nephrogenic fibrosing dermopathy and review of the literature. Semin Arthritis Rheum. 2006;35:238–49.
30. Gibson SE, Farver CF, Prayson RA. Multiorgan involvement in nephrogenic fibrosing dermopathy: an autopsy case and review of the literature. Arch Pathol Lab Med. 2006;130:209–12.
31. Shellock FG, Spinazzi A. MRI safety update 2008: Part 1, MRI contrast agents and nephrogenic systemic fibrosis. Am J Roentgenol. 2008;191:1–11.

32. Knopp EA, Cowper SE. Nephrogenic systemic fibrosis: early recognition and treatment. Semin Dial. 2008;21:123–8. doi:10.1111/j.1525-139X.2007.00399.x.
33. Rydahl C, Thomsen HS, Marckmann P. High prevalence of nephrogenic systemic fibrosis in chronic renal failure patients exposed to gadodiamide, a gadolinium-containing magnetic resonance contrast agent. Invest Radiol. 2008;43:141–4.
34. Todd DJ, Kagan A, Chibnik LB, Kay J. Cutaneous changes of nephrogenic systemic fibrosis: Predictor of early mortality and association with gadolinium exposure. Arthritis Rheum. 2007;56(10):3433–41.
35. Shibui K, Kataoka H, Sato N, Watanabe Y, Kohara M, Mochizuki T. A case of NSF attributable to contrast MRI repeated in a patient with Stage 3 CKD at a renal function of eGFR > 30 mL/min/1.73 m2. Jpn J Nephrol. 2009;51:676.
36. Broome DR. Nephrogenic systemic fibrosis associated with gadolinium based contrast agents: a summary of the medical literature reporting. Eur J Radiol. 2008;66:230–4.
37. Dean PB. Fetal uptake of an intravascular radiologic contrast medium. Rofo. 1977;127:267–70.
38. Kanal E, Barkovich AJ, Bell C, et al. ACR guidance document for safe MR practices: 2007. AJR Am J Roentgenol. 2007;188:1447–74.
39. Panigel M, Wolf G, Zeleznick A. Magnetic resonance imaging of the placenta in rhesus monkeys, Macaca mulatta. J Med Primatol. 1988;17:3–18.
40. Ilett KF, Hackett LP, Paterson JW, McCormick CC. Excretion of metrizamide in milk. Br J Radiol. 1981;54:537–8.
41. Johansen JG. Assessment of a non-ionic contrast medium (Amipaque) in the gastrointestinal tract. Invest Radiol. 1978;13:523–7.
42. Kubik-Huch RA, Gottstein-Aalame NM, Frenzel T, et al. Gadopentetate dimeglumine excretion into human breast milk during lactation. Radiology. 2000;216:555–8.
43. Nielsen ST, Matheson I, Rasmussen JN, Skinnemoen K, Andrew E, Hafsahl G. Excretion of iohexol and metrizoate in human breast milk. Acta Radiol. 1987;28:523–6.
44. Rofsky NM, Weinreb JC, Litt AW. Quantitative analysis of gadopentetate dimeglumine excreted in breast milk. J Magn Reson Imaging. 1993;3:131–2.

Chapter 2
Neurological Imaging

Pallav N. Shah

Introduction

The early 1900s marked the beginning of a new field in imaging, neuroradiology. Skull radiographs became available to the medical community in the first decade of the twentieth century. Ventriculography and pneumoencephalography soon followed 2 decades later. In the ensuing years, intra-arterial catheter-based vascular imaging heralded carotid angiography. Over the next 40 years, many technical advances were made with angiographic imaging; however, patients did not always tolerate these semi-invasive procedures and suffered significant morbidity.

The real breakthrough in neuroimaging occurred with the introduction of computed tomography (CT) imaging in 1971. Soon thereafter, procedures such as ventriculography and pneumoencephalography became obsolete. The revolution in radiology continued with the introduction of magnetic resonance imaging (MRI) in the early 1980s. Noninvasive CT and MR angiography (CTA and MRA) are now the preferred first tests in vascular imaging. Since their inception, they have curtailed the use of conventional intra-arterial catheter-based angiography, which is now typically reserved for therapeutic procedures. Physiologic imaging, utilizing a hybrid of CT, MR, and positron emission tomography (PET) imaging modalities, now complements and at times eclipses traditional morphologic imaging. Today, functional imaging is proving to be an invaluable clinical tool for treatment and pre-surgical planning of many oncology and epilepsy patients.

Today, there are many imaging options available to the neuroradiologist as well as the referring clinician when confronted with a patient with a neurological deficit. Thus, prior to choosing an imaging modality, the pertinent clinical questions must be well-formulated. This means that it is important to conduct a thorough review of

P.N. Shah, M.D. (✉)
Division of Neuroradiology, Department of Radiology, Temple University Hospital, 3401 North Broad Street, Philadelphia, PA 19140, USA
e-mail: pallav.shah@tuhs.temple.edu

W.R. Reinus (ed.), *Clinician's Guide to Diagnostic Imaging*,
DOI 10.1007/978-1-4614-8769-2_2, © Springer Science+Business Media New York 2014

the patient's signs and symptoms. From here the process continues by choosing the appropriate imaging modality, typically X-ray, ultrasound, CT, MR, PET, or conventional angiography. When requesting CT or MRI, the question of whether or not the patient should receive an intravenous contrast agent also needs to be addressed.

Besides clinical indication, other key questions need to be addressed in choosing an imaging examination. What are the risks and benefits of the chosen imaging modality? How will the study alter patient management? Will the patient be able to cooperate fully for the exam? Are there any contraindications to any particular type of imaging? Which imaging modality will yield the greatest amount of information and which be the most cost-effective?

Unfortunately, many disease entities have overlapping clinical presentations and even imaging findings. Hence, choosing the single most appropriate study may prove to be quite difficult. Even so, the correct imaging examination often provides new information that reveals the acuity of the pathology and ultimately determines patient management. In certain situations, imaging allows the clinician to further direct the patient to surgical or medical therapy.

CNS Imaging Modalities: Overview

Plain Film Radiography

Radiographs can be inexpensive and quickly obtained, but the information that they provide is indirect and limited compared with more advanced modalities. Today they play a limited role in central nervous system (CNS) imaging. There remain, however, several key areas where the role of radiographs has not been eclipsed by more advanced imaging techniques. For example, X-rays still remain the primary means for screening patients to exclude metallic foreign bodies that are incompatible with MRI. Plain radiography can be utilized for the evaluation of minor maxillofacial trauma, periodontal disease, surveying the axial and appendicular skeleton for multiple myeloma and screening children for possible child abuse. In addition, radiographs are still used as the first line of imaging in patient with back pain. Flexion and extension spine X-rays still provide the surgeon with valuable functional information when assessing traumatic or degenerative spinal instability. Spondylosis, spondylolisthesis, and spondylolysis can be quickly ruled "in" or "out" using plain radiography.

Plain radiography is often the initial study when assessing for ventricular shunt integrity. Programmable shunt catheter settings and intracranial pressure measurments can be obtained with simple skull radiographs. Plain film imaging continues to play a role in extracranial imaging particularly in the evaluation of dental disease. However, most would agree that CT provides much greater sensitivity and specificity when assessing for intra-calvarial pathology and calvarial, orbital, and maxillofacial trauma.

Although CT and MRI have eclipsed plain film radiography (PFR) for evaluation of the head and maxillofacial region, radiography is often the first line of imaging in screening for spondylosis and related spine disorders. Spine radiographic studies typically include AP, oblique, and lateral views, followed by flexion and extension views to assess for fixed or dynamic instability if needed.

Computed Tomography

Computed tomography (CT) imaging is the most widely used modality in neuroimaging. Its high contrast resolution allows clear delineation of fluid, air, soft tissue, and osseous structures. CT's universal availability and accessibility at all hours of the day is often the primary reason for selecting it over MRI, particularly in the acute setting. CT permits sequential imaging of the head and neck region within seconds. Rapid imaging and multi-planar reconstruction capabilities allow quick diagnosis of surgical emergencies in acutely ill patients. Furthermore, it has higher accuracy for diagnosing acute intracranial hemorrhage than MRI. Subacutely, it provides an accurate means to reevaluate ICU patients for interval change in CNS pathology. This is particularly useful in patients who have Glasgow Coma Scale (GCS) scores below <8. Non-contrast imaging is recommended in the evaluation of patients with trauma.

In general, IV contrast should be used when there is concern for infection or neoplastic disease. Contrast administration also allows CT to depict neurovascular anatomy from the aortic arch to the dural venous sinuses in minutes. In addition, CT's ability to rapidly and repeatedly scan a large volume of tissue allows perfusion imaging after a dose of intravenous contrast.

Despite the tremendous benefits to CT imaging, one of its main drawbacks is its use of ionizing radiation. This has raised concern of an increased long-term risk of cancer, particularly in young patients [1]. With collaboration among physicists, imaging vendors, and radiologists, new imaging recommendations are now available that reduce radiation dose for both pediatric and adult patients. Nationwide campaigns such as Image Gently and Image Wisely provide radiologists alternative strategies to reduce radiation exposure without significantly decreasing imaging quality.

Ultrasound

Sonographic imaging (ultrasound, US) plays a very specific role in CNS imaging. In the pediatric population, sonography is used to assess in utero malformations and perinatal complications such as germinal matrix hemorrhage with or without hydrocephalus. Prior to complete ossification of the spine, US can also be used to screen for and diagnose neural tube defects such as meningoceles, myelomeningoceles, and spina bifida. Better anatomical detail and superior soft tissue contrast resolution is available with MRI, but in younger patients anesthesia may be required for the patient to tolerate the time necessary for an MR.

Trans Cranial Doppler imaging provides a real time, dynamic bedside evaluation of intracranial arterial vasospasm. This noninvasive, quick, and readily available test can be tremendously helpful to the neurosurgeon in identifying vasospasm during the critical period after subarachnoid hemorrhage.

The largest indication for ultrasound in CNS imaging is carotid stenosis. This is a quick reliable noninvasive method of screening patients with carotid atherosclerotic disease, symptomatic or not, for carotid stenosis. Ultrasound's main drawback is that it is operator-dependent. Therefore, a poorly performed examination can lead to an incorrect diagnosis. Newer, 3D sonographic imaging and video capture technology allows the radiologist to provide a more "real time" evaluation and lessens the concern over operator dependence.

Magnetic Resonance Imaging

Since its initial clinical use in the 1980s, MR scanning equipment and imaging sequences have greatly improved and now provide exquisite anatomic detail and soft tissue characterization. MRI, like CT, can obtain multi-planar modality image sets, but without the use of ionizing radiation. It has allowed both better diagnosis and better understanding of CNS pathology. MR brain imaging is superior to CT imaging particularly when assessing the posterior fossa structures and also in evaluating the meninges and cranial nerves. In spine imaging, it is able to assess bone marrow abnormalities, define and grade osseous and discogenic spondylosis, and provide excellent gray and white matter cord distinction.

Time of flight (TOF) MRI techniques can also be used to perform vascular imaging, with or without contrast, using maximum intensity projection and multi-planar reconstruction. This is particularly useful in the evaluation of the Circle of Willis for aneurysms, arterial occlusions, and arteriovenous malformations (AVMs). In addition, TOF imaging can quantify and also localize atherosclerotic disease and vascular injury. Dural venous flow can also be studied with MRI utilizing either TOF or phase contrast scanning techniques.

MRI is by far the preferred modality, particularly in the subacute setting because of its superior soft tissue resolution and contrast. Its lack of "around the clock" availability unfortunately prevents it from being more widely used, especially in the acute setting. Additional drawbacks also include multiple contraindications, some of which are absolute while others are relative (Table 1.3, Chap. 1). Patients who are claustrophobic may not be able to tolerate imaging because of the configuration of the scanner. More recently, the concern for nephrogenic systemic fibrosis (NSF) has also precluded utilization of contrast MRI in selected patient groups.

Clinical Scenarios

Headache (Pediatric)

Headache is a very common complaint in children [2, 3]. The majority of pediatric headaches are benign. Headaches in general, and particularly the migraine type, are more common among adolescent females. Studies show that CNS imaging of pediatric patients yields a significant positive finding only 1 % of the time [4, 5]. Rarely, an underlying brain tumor or other structural abnormality is the etiology of the headaches in pediatric patients with an annual incidence of 0.3 % of patients [6]. The high prevalence of headaches and the low yield of pathology detected at imaging raise the question of whether there is a need to expose pediatric patients with "isolated" headaches to radiation or whether it is wise to devote healthcare resources to this end. Many studies have tried to define associated signs or symptoms that may yield a higher rate of structural pathology in children with headaches.

Retrospective data from the Childhood Brain Tumor Consortium suggests that neurologic deficits and/or papilledema herald underlying structural brain pathology. Neurologic deficits include gait disturbance, abnormal reflexes, nystagmus, confusion, cranial nerve findings, and altered sensation. Headaches of increasing frequency, duration, or intensity should raise suspicion for an underlying structural lesion. An intense, prolonged, and incapacitating headache in the absence of migraines is also concerning for underlying pathology.

A "thunderclap" headache, which is severe headache of acute onset, is most commonly reported in adults but also occurs in children. These headaches classically correlate with imaging findings of subarachnoid hemorrhage (SAH) and intracranial hemorrhage that arise from a precipitous rupture of an aneurysm or AVM. Carotid or vertebral dissection has been associated with sudden onset of severe unilateral headache and accompanying neurologic findings in pediatric patients.

Neuroimaging with a non-contrast CT scan has been advocated for patients with sudden onset of a severe headache, particularly in the absence of a family history of migraines [7]. If CT imaging reveals subarachnoid or parenchymal hemorrhage, further evaluation for aneurysm or vascular malformation must be performed, using either CT angiography (CTA) or MRA. CTA is more widely available and is quicker than MRA, but carries risk from radiation exposure. If these noninvasive methods fail to show a lesion, conventional catheter-based angiography should be considered. Catheter angiography not only provides more definitive information regarding a vascular lesion but also offers the option of immediate intra-arterial and/or intravenous therapy.

Typically, migraine headaches can be distinguished from other types of headaches by history. Patients whose migraine headaches are associated with an initial aura may also have symptoms such as unilateral numbness and tingling, or transient hemiplegia, aphasia, and/or apraxia. Thus, clinicians may have difficulty distinguishing the first few episodes of migraine headaches from other more ominous CNS pathology such as brain tumor, SAH, vasculopathy, or AVM.

This concern may lead to imaging before the clinical diagnosis and pattern of migraine headaches is established or recognized. One of the distinguishing features of migraine headaches is their temporal nature. Neurologic findings in migraine headaches are fleeting while deficits from brain tumors usually persist. Children, in particular, are symptom-free between episodes of migraines. Most clinicians do not advocate imaging in patients with an established diagnosis of classic or common migraine [7]. There is no supportive data for imaging patients who either have nonprogressive migraine headaches, or who have a positive family history [8, 9].

Complicated migraines are defined as those with associated focal neurologic deficit. The presentation of a complicated migraine often overlaps the presentation of headache caused by a brain tumor. Imaging is therefore recommended in these cases to exclude the latter [8, 9]. Patients with ophthalmologic migraines may present with unilateral ptosis or complete third nerve palsy. This often can be confused with a structural CNS abnormality, and therefore imaging may be beneficial.

Sinogenic headaches, i.e., headaches caused by sinus pathology, occur in both children and adults. Although the diagnosis of acute sinusitis is made clinically, complaints of persistent and severe headache as the dominant feature of sinusitis are worrisome. In these cases, imaging is indicated to exclude intracranial extension of disease. Signs or symptoms that provoke concern for intracranial extension include high fever, confusion, and change in mental status with or without focal signs. Intracranial spread of infection causes dural irritation and localized encephalitis which in turn causes headache.

Suppurative intracranial collections between the skull and dura are less prevalent in children than adolescents. These empyemas most commonly arise via extension of paranasal sinus disease. Imaging with either CT or MRI plays a key role in characterizing the intracranial pathology as meningitis, encephalitis, or meningoencephalitis and showing the presence of hemorrhage/infarction or brain abscess. Contrast is recommended as it enhances the conspicuousness of a subtle collection. MRI is preferable for diagnosing epidural empyemas because it has the ability to distinguish among different types of fluid [10].

Headaches associated with fever or known systemic illnesses may indicate possible meningitis or encephalitis. Altered consciousness, nuchal rigidity, or other neurological signs also indicate a need for neuroimaging. In addition, some diseases, including neoplasms and/or systemic illnesses such as sickle cell disease or hypertension or those that cause immune compromise, predispose patients to intracranial pathology. In high-risk groups such as these, the presence of a severe or unremitting headache may herald significant intracranial pathology and indicate the need for imaging. In immune-compromised pediatric patients particularly, the threshold for imaging should be low.

In summary, neuroimaging generally is not warranted for patients with primary, e.g., migraine or chronic, headaches but usually is indicated for secondary headaches, i.e., those associated with underlying pathology. Headache characteristics, the patient's medical history, and neurological examination findings distinguish the headache as primary or secondary. Patients presenting with secondary headaches in urgent clinical situations require emergent CT while MRI is preferable in nonurgent situations. Emergent CT examination is recommended for patients presenting with sudden, severe "thunderclap" headaches or complaining of the "worst headache in their life."

Headache (Adult)

Several clinical indicators have been studied to determine when neuroimaging is needed in adults. Most of this data come from studies on patients who visit the emergency department (ED) with a chief complaint of headache [11–13]. Indications include focal neurologic deficit, alteration in the character of the headache, persistence of headache despite analgesics, abrupt onset, and increasing frequency and intensity of the headache. Of these, abrupt onset and focal neurologic findings most strongly predicted intracranial lesions. Overall, 36 % of the patients who present with a headache as well as a focal neurologic deficit had significant pathology on imaging [14]. Another study showed that ED patients with a chief complaint of headache who also had decreased level of consciousness, paralysis, or papilledema were most likely to have visible CT or MT imaging pathology. In this study, 35 % of those who presented with headache and a positive neurologic exam had intracranial pathology shown by imaging [15]. Another study of ED patients with a chief complaint of headache who had neuroimaging, either CT or cerebral angiography, again showed that an abnormal neurologic examination was most significantly correlated with positive imaging findings [16].

Information concerning the workup of headaches in the ambulatory setting is limited. In this group about 3 % of outpatients presenting to their physician with a new headache undergo CT evaluation [17]. Of these, only 4 % of the scans reveal a significant finding and/or treatable lesion [18]. Expert guidelines for headaches among the ambulatory population recommend neuroimaging for migraine patients only in the presence of persistent focal abnormal neurological findings. They note inadequate evidence for recommending neuroimaging for patients with tension type headaches. They also note inadequate evidence for or against neuroimaging for headache in the presence or absence of non-focal symptoms such as dizziness, syncope, nausea, lack of coordination, the "worst headache ever," headache that awakens the patient from sleep, and increasing frequency of headaches [19]. The radiologic literature supports imaging in the setting papilledema, meningismus, partial seizure, increase in pain with coughing, sneezing, or change in body position, and any new headache in an HIV-positive patient [20, 21].

When confronted with a patient who complains of headache, the quality, location, duration, and time course of the headache and the conditions that produce, exacerbate, or relieve it should be carefully reviewed. Information regarding the patient's medical and family history also should be taken into consideration. This clinical data may provide clues to the underlying cause of headache so that a judicious decision can be made for neuroimaging either with CT or MR (Fig. 2.1).

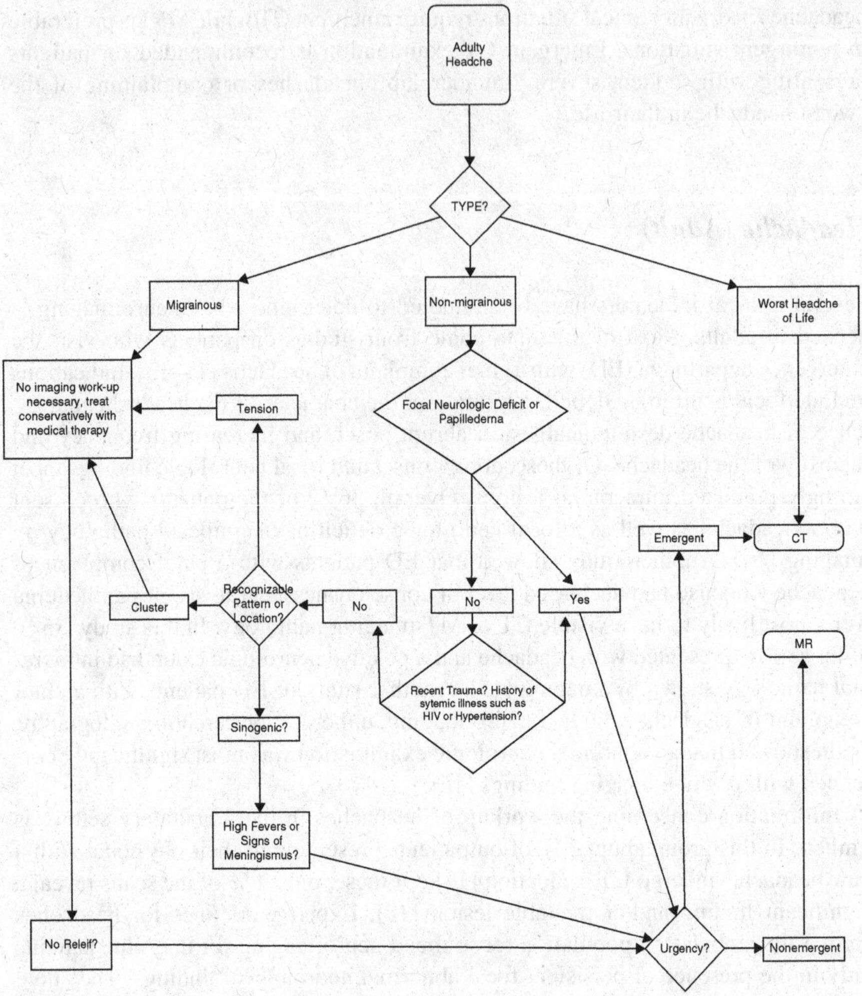

Fig. 2.1 Algorithmic approach to Imaging for patients presenting with headache

Seizure

A seizure is a finite event of altered cerebral function because of excessive and abnormal electrical activity within the brain. Epilepsy is a chronic condition which predisposes the patient to repeated seizures. It has been estimated that one out of eight individuals will experience at least one seizure in their lifetime [22].

The International League Against Epilepsy reclassified epileptic seizures in 2010 in an effort to improve diagnosis, treatment, and management of patients who live with this chronic illness (Fig. 2.2). They classified seizures as generalized or focal

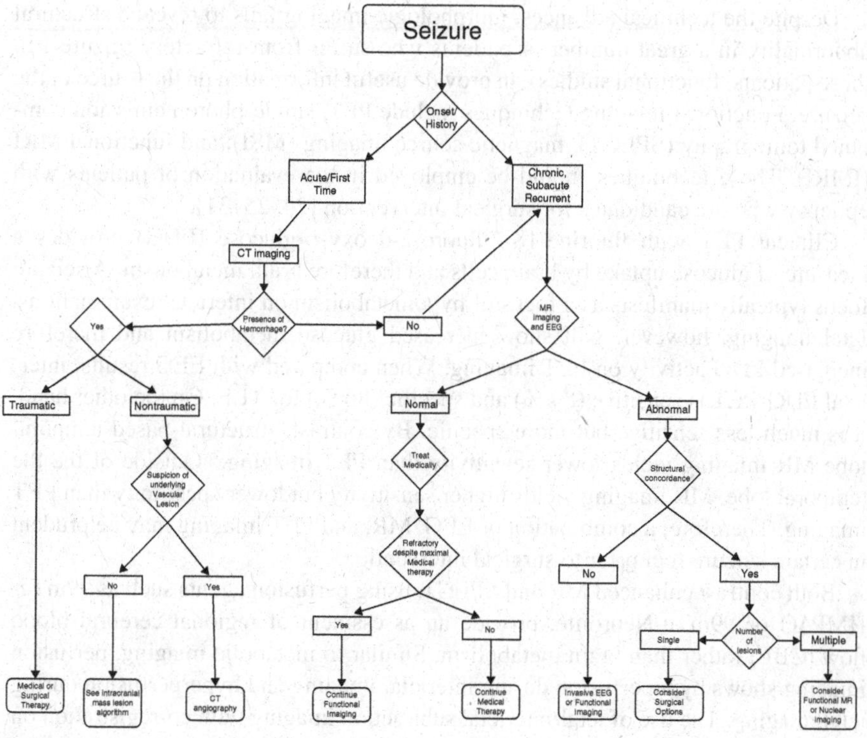

Fig. 2.2 Algorithmic approach to imaging for patients presenting with seizure

and then further subdivided them into tonic-clonic, absence, myoclonic, clonic, tonic, and atonic types. The distinction between "focal" and "generalized" seizures is important because it reflects the extent of abnormal brain activity. Generalized seizures rapidly affect both cerebral hemispheres and both sides of the body, even when they are caused by a "focal" lesion. Certain types of seizure disorders are more likely than others to be associated with structural brain lesions such as tumors, infection, infarction, traumatic brain injury, vascular malformations, and developmental abnormalities. Therefore, knowledge of the type of a patient's seizure helps to determine when neuroimaging is clinically indicated and what type of study is appropriate.

Given the superior soft tissue contrast and multi-planar capability of MRI, it is easy to understand why it provides the highest sensitivity and accuracy when assessing virtually any cause of epilepsy. MR can provide high-resolution structural imaging in epilepsy with either 1.5 or 3.0 T MR scanners, including tailored thin section imaging through the mesial temporal lobes in cases of temporal lobe epilepsy (TLE). In these patients, MR imaging can demonstrate hippocampal atrophy, subtle signal alterations, certain structural abnormalities accompanying cortical dysplasias, hamartomas, and/or other developmental abnormalities. Anatomic imaging identifies a focal abnormality in as many as half of all patients with focal seizures [23].

Despite the technical advances, morphologic imaging fails to reveal a structural abnormality in a great number of patients who suffer from refractory seizures. In these patients, functional studies can provide useful information on the source of the seizure. Functional imaging techniques include PET, single-photon emission computed tomography (SPECT), magnetic source imaging (MSI), and functional MRI (fMRI). These techniques should be employed in the evaluation of patients with epilepsy who are candidates for surgical intervention [24, 25–31].

Clinical PET with fluorine-18-2-fluoro-2-deoxy-D-glucose (FDG) provides a measure of glucose uptake by brain cells and therefore brain metabolism. A seizure focus typically manifests as a focus of hypometabolism on interictal examinations. Ictal imaging, however, will show increased glucose metabolism and therefore increased FDG activity on PET imaging. When compared with EEG results, interictal FDG-PET is sensitive (84 %) and specific (86 %) for TLE. On the other hand, it is much less sensitive but more specific. By contrast, structural-based temporal lobe MR imaging yields lower sensitivity than PET imaging. Outside of the the temporal lobe, MR imaging yields higher sensitivity but lower specificity than PET imaging. Therefore, a combination of EEG, MR, and PET imaging may be prudent in certain seizure foci prior to surgical intervention.

Both contrast enhanced MR and SPECT, using perfusion agents such as 99mTc-HMPAO or 99mTc-Neurolite, provide an assessment of regional cerebral blood flow (CBF) rather than brain metabolism. Similar to metabolic imaging, perfusion imaging shows hypoperfusion during interictal imaging and hyperperfusion during ictal imaging. The use of ictal/interictal subtraction imaging with co-registration on MRI and image-guided surgery datasets is proving to be more useful than interictal imaging alone [32, 33]. Unfortunately, the need to inject the blood flow agent within 90 seconds of the seizure for the ictal phase of imaging is often an insurmountable technological challenge.

fMRI techniques include phosphorus and proton spectroscopy (MRS), perfusion, and blood oxygen level-dependent (BOLD) activation. Widespread availability of fMRI imaging is limited because this technique requires specialized MR scanners that can perform and then post-process fast echo-planar pulse sequences. MRS provides in-vivo chemical analysis of the brain. It shows differential metabolite values in epileptogenic regions of the brain compared to normal brain parenchyma. MRS is used as an adjunct pre-surgical examination for seizure source localization in difficult cases of extra-temporal and partial epilepsy. It reduces the need for invasive intracranial electroencephalography (iEEG) recordings.

Both EEG and magnetoencephalography (MEG) offer significantly higher temporal resolution than PET, SPECT, and fMRI. Recent improvements in MEG technology allow complete brain coverage. MEG is utilized in preoperative evaluation of patients with intractable or medically refractory seizures [34, 35]. The MEG images are often superimposed on high-resolution MR images. MEG is not a "front-line" tool for evaluation of epilepsy, but may be used in select patients who: (a) are surgical candidates for resection, (b) do not have an MR demonstrable lesion or have multiple potential seizure foci, or (c) might otherwise require invasive monitoring (iEEG). MEG is thus complimentary to EEG and may confirm lesions seen on MRI as the source of the seizure. MEG provides better spatial resolution compared with EEG [35] and can also guide the placement of iEEG grids. In certain patients it may also help to discern important seizure foci among multiple potential seizure foci suggested by other tests.

Focal Neurologic Deficit

A focal neurologic deficit is a collection of symptoms or signs that can be attributed to a specific anatomic site in the CNS. A dedicated neurologic examination often can define the CNS source of the deficit. In some cases, however, the etiology of the abnormality may be difficult to define, and in these cases imaging can narrow differential diagnostic considerations. Image interpretation can be much more sensitive and specific if the radiologist is made aware of the onset (acute vs. insidious) as well as temporal behavior (stable, worsening, or resolving) of the focal neurologic deficit.

In general, acute onset of a focal neurologic deficit implies a vascular etiology while a more insidious onset or a chronic process suggests an underlying mass lesion (Fig. 2.3). CT imaging can be used to screen patients for suspected infarction, but is often insensitive in the hyper-acute setting. At times, certain subtle CT findings such as an obscured insular ribbon or hyperattenuation of the middle cerebral artery can be the first imaging clue to the location as well as severity of the stroke on early CT. Diffusion weighted MR imaging (DWI) is much more sensitive than CT in detecting acute ischemia-induced cytotoxic edema and thus the specific brain tissue at risk. The main goal of CT in the setting of acute infarction is to exclude intracranial hemorrhage in patients who might otherwise be candidates for thrombolytic therapy. Contrast administration is not necessary with either CT or MR when evaluating for acute infarction.

Besides ischemic events, parenchymal or SAH also may cause an acute focal neurologic deficit. Non-contrast CT imaging is the preferred technique for screening for acute intracranial hemorrhage because of wide availability, short scan time, and high sensitivity for detecting acute hemorrhage [36, 37]. While MR is sensitive for detecting and differentiating acute from chronic blood products, it is generally not as available in the acute setting.

A slowly progressive focal neurologic deficit generally implies the presence of an expanding and evolving intracranial lesion such as a primary or metastatic neoplasm. Conversely, a more subacute presentation typically correlates with an infectious process. While CT is invaluable for screening for either infection or neoplasm acutely, a contrast enhanced MR study will provide far more anatomic detail, define the extent of disease, and allow for soft tissue characterization.

Transient Ischemic Attack

Over the past decade, there has been considerable debate over the definition of transient ischemic attack (TIA), particularly the acceptable duration of the transient symptomatology. Conventionally, TIA was defined as a focal neurologic deficit

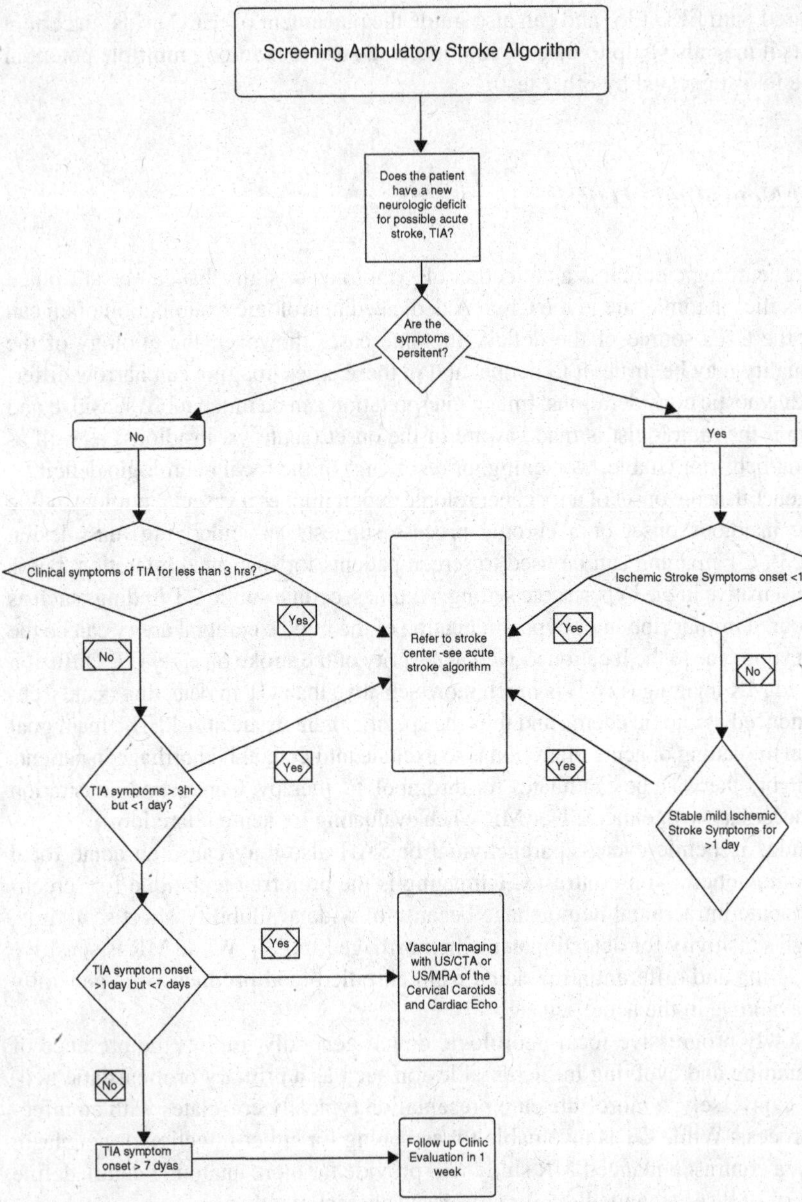

Fig. 2.3 Algorithmic approach to imaging patients who present with a focal neurologic deficit in the ambulatory setting: screening for acute stroke

lasting less than 24 h. The problem with a time-based definition is that it does not adequately identify patients who may benefit from thrombolytic therapy (rtPA, recombinant tissue plasminogen activator). A tissue-based definition is preferable because although most (70 %) TIA symptoms last for 2 h or less, many of these patients (30–50 %) show tissue injury on diffusion weighted MRI (DWI) [38–40]. The American Stroke Association has recently proposed a new definition of TIA as "a transient episode of neurologic dysfunction caused by focal brain, spinal cord, or retinal ischemia, without acute infarction" [39, 41]. Based on the current FDA recommendations, however, only the presence of acute hemorrhage on non-contrast CT (NCCT) is a contraindication to rtPA treatment in the first 3 h after the onset of deficit. Even rapidly improving symptoms in the first 3 h and no DWI changes on MR may not justify withholding rtPA because as many as a third of these patients go on to subsequent severe deterioration if left untreated.

In addition, 10–15 % of all strokes are heralded by a TIA within 90 days—half of these within 48 h. Thus, a history of recent TIA should trigger an immediate workup for stroke risks and additional tissue and vascular imaging studies [39, 42, 43]. These imaging studies typically begin with non-contrast CT, followed by MR and carotid Doppler US to identify a possible source of thromboembolic disease.

Stroke

As noted above, NCCT has been the preferred modality for initial imaging of suspected stroke because it is widely available and very sensitive for acute hemorrhage. CT effectively detects acute hemorrhage in brain parenchyma and in the subarachnoid, subdural, and intraventricular spaces. Unfortunately, it is insensitive at detecting acute ischemic tissue injury. Recent development of computed tomographic perfusion (CTP) imaging has increased sensitivity for detection of acute cerebrovascular-induced tissue damage. While CTP imaging requires contrast, magnetic resonance perfusion (MRP) imaging may be performed with or without contrast.

CT perfusion studies are performed by rapidly imaging and reimaging a target region of the brain immediately following contrast bolus. The technique is based on the central volume principle which states that CBF is equivalent to the cerebral blood volume (CBV) divided by the mean transit time (MTT). Both CTP and MRP imaging can measure CBV, CBF, time to peak (TTP), and MTT. Quantitative and qualitative measurement of these parameters provides a method of assessing regional tissue perfusion to identify relative regions of ischemia or infarction. In general, a CBF of 10–15 mL/100 g/min or less is considered infarcted tissue whereas a rate of 15–20 mL/100 g/min is considered ischemic. Any region of tissue that is under-perfused, but not infracted, surrounding infracted tissue is considered the penumbra. Alternatively the penumbra can also be considered as a volume of low blood flow tissue that is larger than the infarcted volume by 20 % or more. Relative "mismatch" of tissue flow and volume compared with the centrally infracted core tissue, in the absence of acute hemorrhage, indicates brain tissue that may be salvaged with the use of thrombolytic therapy. Technically, MRP has several advantages over CTP. It does not use ionizing radiation, has less risk of renal toxicity, known contrast reactions, and does not cause fluid overload compared to iodinated contrast materials. MRP has less variability than CTP quantitative methods [44], and, unlike CT, MRI can measure directly cellular viability using diffusion restriction techniques. It also can assess a larger volume of brain tissue than CTP. The newer generation of CT scanners, with their larger number of detector arrays, is decreasing the volume gap between techniques, however [45]. Despite these advantages, the wide availability of CT and the rapidity with which it can be performed in a limited 3 h clinical onset window mitigates the advantages of MR. Given the abovementioned risks and benefits of imaging, an appropriate plan of care can be rapidly implemented to diagnose, define, and possibly treat a patient presenting with an acute stroke (Fig. 2.4).

Role of Imaging in Specific Scenarios

Carotid Stenosis

In recent years, the medical community has made a concerted effort to reduce the incidence of stroke by identifying patients most at risk. Much effort has been expended to identify risk factors for atherosclerotic disease, and new strategies have been developed to reduce the rate of stroke in high-risk patients [46]. Efforts range from modification of lifestyle to preemptive surgical or endovascular carotid artery intervention. Randomized, prospective clinical trials that include imaging and other criteria have shown that surgical endarterectomy is effective in reducing stroke morbidity of both asymptomatic and symptomatic patients [47–52].

Imaging today offers a number of sensitive, noninvasive and therefore low risk, tests, all directed at diagnosing the most common cause of a stroke—carotid artery atherosclerosis—in "at risk" patient groups such as those with a carotid bruit [53, 54]. While duplex ultrasound (US) and computed tomography angiography (CTA), magnetic resonance angiography (MRA) and time-resolved contrast enhanced MRA (CE-MRA) all have high diagnostic accuracies for detecting internal carotid stenosis, 70–99 % [55, 56], only US appears to offer cost-effective initial screening. However, given the operator imaging variability with sonography as well as the artifact created from calcified plaques, and the difficulty in distinguishing subtotal from total occlusion, a full endorsement of its routine use as the sole examination before endarterectomy cannot be made [55, 57]. Most radiologists today recommend combined use of US with CE-MRA [53–55, 57–59].

Multi-slice CTA offers an alternative means of examination; however, it poses risks from intravenous iodinated contrast administration. CTA requires a large intravenous contrast injection volume and hence has the potential for contrast-induced nephrotoxicity or anaphylaxis. In addition, CT exposes the patient to an ionizing radiation dose. CTA also may be less accurate at evaluating the degree of luminal narrowing in the presence of calcified plaque than some other techniques [56, 60, 61].

It is hoped that better plaque characterization will improve the predictive value of imaging at identifying clinically significant carotid stenosis for patients with

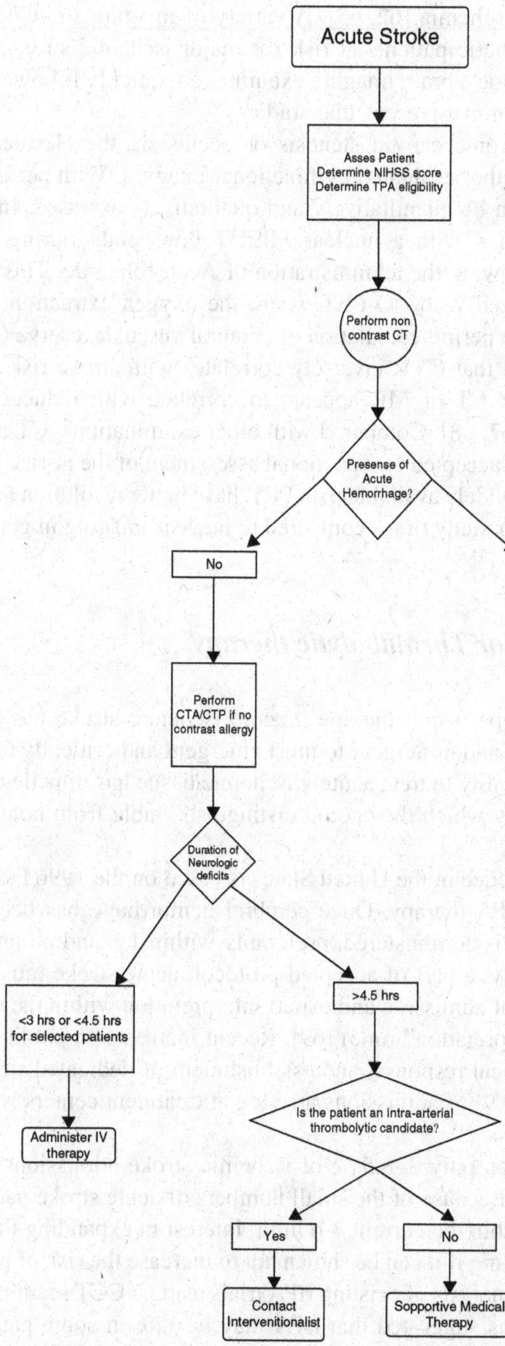

Fig. 2.4 Algorithmic approach for imaging and treatment of acute stroke

symptomatic cerebral ischemia [62, 63]. A variety of imaging strategies could be undertaken in symptomatic patients at risk for major ischemic stroke, where the initial study could include a brain imaging examination, quickly followed by one of the abovementioned noninvasive vascular studies.

In patients with chronic carotid stenosis or occlusion, the elevated ischemic stroke risk could be further evaluated by functional imaging. With perfusion imaging, CBV and CBF can be quantitatively and qualitatively assessed. In the recent past, this was performed with a nuclear SPECT flow study during a rest and "challenge" phase following the administration of Acetazolamide. This same principle also can be utilized with ^{15}O-PET where the oxygen extraction differences pre- and post-challenge permit calculation of cerebral vascular reserve (CVR) [64–66]. It has been shown that CVR inversely correlates with stroke risk. Low CBV measurement by either CT or MR appears to correlate with reduced CVR and increased stroke risk [67, 68]. Compared with other examinations, CT and MR are becoming more widely accepted for functional assessment of the at-risk brain tissue because they are more widely available than PET, have better resolution than SPECT, and have overall shorter study times compared to nuclear imaging in general.

Triaging Patients for Thrombolytic therapy

Since the advent of reperfusion therapies, acute ischemic stroke has been transformed from incurable and nonurgent to most emergent and critically treatable. As discussed above, the ability to treat acutely ischemic tissue has impelled physicians to develop a method by which they could distinguish viable from nonviable brain parenchyma.

Current clinical practice in the United States is based on the 1996 FDA approval of intravenous (IV) rtPA therapy. Once cerebral hemorrhage has been excluded using NCCT, the drug is administered, preferably within 1 h and no later than 3 h after symptom onset. As a part of accepted protocol, acute stroke must obtain the NCCT within 25 min of admission and expert interpretation within the next 20 min (45 min "door-to-interpretation" time) [69]. Recent increases in public awareness, faster emergency medical response, and establishment of dedicated stroke centers have resulted in 19–60 % of admissions arriving at treatment centers within 3 h of symptom onset.

Despite these efforts, only 3–8.5 % of ischemic stroke admissions qualify for rtPA therapy [70–72]. Because of the small numbers of acute stroke patients qualifying for treatment within the current 3-h limit, interest in expanding the treatment window has been growing if it can be shown not to increase the risk of hemorrhage. A pooled risk-benefit analysis of existing rtPA trials using NCCT scan for the exclusion of hemorrhage has suggested that rtPA may be safe in some patients out to 4.5 h after stroke, but the FDA and ASA recommendations have not yet been modified to include this expanded treatment window in published guidelines.

The American College of Radiology (ACR) appropriateness criteria may change in the very near future as the results of these studies and trials become conclusive.

There is growing evidence that intra-arterial (IA) thrombolytic delivery and mechanical clot extraction methods are beneficial either alone or with IV rtPA therapy in patients who fall outside the 3-h limit or who have large-vessel occlusion or larger clot burden. They may be at a higher risk of hemorrhage, however. Furthermore, complexities of organizing these later stage therapies have limited their widespread adoption in general [73–75, 76].

Many centers now routinely perform CT perfusion, but currently there is no clear consensus on whether the information obtained from CTP should be used to guide intravenous (IV) or intra-arterial (IA) therapy. MR perfusion and diffusion imaging could be performed instead, but unfortunately this technique is time-prohibitive and not universally available on a 24 h/7days a week basis. Furthermore, contraindications listed previously (Table 1.3, Chap. 1) may preclude patients from having an MR.

It should be noted that in addition to NCCT to exclude acute hemorrhage in new onset stroke patients, previously described multimodality MRI and CT studies also may be useful to confirm the diagnosis, classify the subtype of stroke, demonstrate lesion location, identify vascular occlusion, and guide other management decisions both within and beyond the 3 h period. Currently, however, ASA and others' guidelines specifically recommend that emergency IV rtPA treatment within the 3 h window not be delayed in order to obtain multimodality imaging studies and furthermore that treatment not be withheld on the basis of either negative or additional positive MR or CT findings, other than acute hemorrhage [77–81].

Intracranial Mass Lesion

While the discovery of an intracranial mass lesion may be incidental, patients can present with focal or non-focal neurologic deficits. Signs or symptoms may range from headaches, seizures, syncope, to change in mental status. Clinical history along with imaging can provide a framework for proper categorization of the disease process. General categories for possible etiologies of an intracranial mass lesion include infectious, inflammatory, traumatic, vascular, or neoplastic. Contrast utilization is often quite helpful not only in characterizing the disease process but also evaluating the full anatomical extent of disease. While the role of imaging initially was limited to providing anatomic details, the present role is to provide functional information through a vast array of modalities such as perfusion, diffusion, MR spectroscopy, and PET [82]. Sophisticated imaging techniques allow insight into such processes as the free movement of water molecules, microvascular integrity, chemical composition, and glucose metabolism of the lesion. Merging the morphologic and functional information gained from these advanced imaging techniques can then provide a more comprehensive assessment of the lesion so that we may better understand its physiology and in turn predict its behavior (Fig. 2.5).

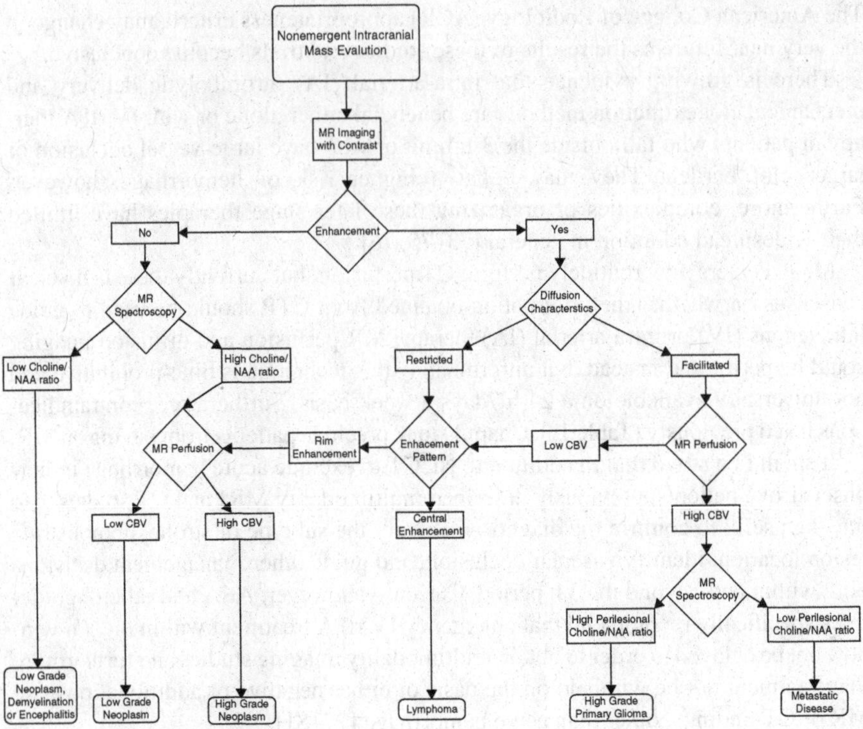

Fig. 2.5 Algorithmic approach for image-based characterization of an intracranial mass lesion

Subarachnoid Hemorrhage

Since CT is highly accurate for the diagnosis of acute hemorrhage, it has been the mainstay in emergent evaluation of acute intracranial bleeding, especially subarachnoid or parenchymal hemorrhage, both of which are associated with high morbidity and mortality [83, 84]. In the case of SAH caused by aneurysms, the high morbidity rate is partly due to a high likelihood of re-bleeding. Early surgical intervention or intravascular coiling is recommended to reduce morbidity. Before therapy can be undertaken, a cerebral angiogram is required to define the aneurysm's location and morphology. Studies show that catheter-based angiography has approximately 90 % sensitivity in detecting an aneurysm. This sensitivity, however, decreases to approximately 80 % in the setting of SAH resulting from small aneurysm size or in the face of aneurysm thrombosis, local vasospasm, or an incomplete study [85, 86]. Traditionally, non-visualization of an aneurysm on the initial scan from any of the above reasons warranted a follow-up catheter-based repeat angiogram 1 week after the initial examination. The clinician should be aware that the cost and risk to obtain the additional 1–2 % diagnostic yield has been debated [87].

Today, clinical practice has shifted toward initial NCCT for SAH detection and if found immediate CTA for aneurysm detection. Studies have shown that CTA has overall detection sensitivities of 85–95 % for aneurysms greater than 2 mm in diameter [88–90]. Today, treatment of intracranial aneurysms following SAH is increasingly based on CTA alone [91, 92]. In addition, the appearance of new neurologic changes suggestive of post-SAH vasospasm, ischemia, or hydrocephalus is increasingly investigated with transcranial Doppler (TCD) and CT imaging with CTA and CTP. Catheter angiography and 123I-IMP SPECT are used less frequently than in the past [85, 93–98].

Aneurysm Screening

In the absence of predisposing risk factors such as family history, polycystic kidney disease, connective tissue disorder, or collagen vascular disease, the need to screen the general population for aneurysms is debated. Proponents raise concerns over the cumulative long-term risk of morbidity and mortality from SAH, particularly for aneurysms larger than 2.5 cm. When this is weighed against the relatively low risk of clipping and coiling unruptured intracranial aneurysms, data suggest that there may be a clinical role for prophylactic aneurysm screening [99, 100]. Those against catheter-based angiographic screening raise concerns about the thromboembolic complication risk from the procedure and argue that screening is not cost-effective. MRA and CTA offer an alternative cost-effective and noninvasive option [95, 101, 102].

To date, individuals with a history of aneurysm or SAH in a first-degree relative have been considered candidates for screening [103]. Screening patients with a positive family history using MRA or CTA may be appropriate, but its impact on patient outcome is questionable thus far [103].

Vascular Malformation

Vascular malformations, including AVM, pial arteriovenous fistulae, and cavernous hemangiomas in younger patients, as well as dural fistulae in older individuals, can give rise to parenchymal hemorrhage. Diagnosis, assessment of risk for future hemorrhage, and effective treatment planning are predicated on the determination of the lesion size, location, pattern of venous drainage, and the presence of an intra-nidal aneurysm [104, 105]. After an acute hemorrhage, patients may be evaluated with intra-arterial angiography. If the case is complicated, MR can provide soft tissue detail and visualization of associated parenchymal injury. Time-resolved dynamic CE-MRA imaging has been utilized to provide a noninvasive option, but its capabilities fall short in the evaluation of high-flow AVMs. It may play a role, however, in follow-up of partially embolized lesions. Baseline and follow-up MR may be useful for incompletely embolized malformations or as a noninvasive, low-risk means of identifying ischemic complications and assessing response to therapy in patients undergoing stereotactic radiosurgery [106]. Currently, only CTA performed using dual-source, flat-panel, and wide-detector scanners provide adequate temporal resolution for noninvasive evaluation of AVM with CT [45, 107].

Treated Aneurysm Follow-Up

Treatment of intracranial aneurysms has evolved in recent years toward greater use of endovascular coil embolization instead of or combined with surgical clipping [87, 108, 109]. Catheter digital subtraction angiography (DSA) is used to identify incomplete occlusion as part of routine follow-up-treated aneurysms. CTA is hampered by star artifact produced by the aneurysm clip and/or coils. Recently, interest has arisen in using TOF MRA for this purpose. Although routine TOF MRI is also prone to artifact from susceptibilty, dephasing, turbulent flow, and T1 saturation signal loss, these shortcomings are being mitigated quickly with newer imaging sequences. Experience on higher field (3 T) MR scanners suggests that TOF MRA, CE-MRA, and post-contrast volumetric techniques compare favorably with catheter DSA [110, 111]. Safety clearance for ferromagnetic devices should be obtained from published sources or device manufacturers before attempting MRI [112].

References

1. Pearce MS, Salotti JA, Little MP, McHugh K, Lee C, Kim KP, Howe NL, Ronckers CM, Rajaraman P, Sir Craft AW, Parker L, Berrington de González A. Radiation exposure from CT scans in childhood and subsequent risk of leukeamia and brain tumours: a retrospective cohort study. Lancet. 2012;380(9840):499–505.
2. Bille BS. Migraine in school children. A study of the incidence and short-term prognosis, and a clinical, psychological and electroencephalographic comparison between children with migraine and matched controls. Acta Paediatr. 1962;51 Suppl 136:1–151.
3. Sillanpaa M. Headache in children. In: Olessen J, editor. Headache classification and epidemiology. New York, NY: Raven; 1994. p. 273–81.
4. Schwedt TJ, Guo Y, Rothner AD. "Benign" imaging abnormalities in children and adolescents with headache. Headache. 2006;46(3):387–98.
5. Sempere AP, Porta-Etessam J, Medrano V, et al. Neuroimaging in the evaluation of patients with non-acute headache. Cephalalgia. 2005;25(1):30–5.
6. The Childhood Brain Tumor Consortium. The epidemiology of headache among children with brain tumor. Headache in children with brain tumors. J Neurooncol. 1991;10(1):31–46.
7. Landtblom AM, Fridriksson S, Boivie J, Hillman J, Johansson G, Johansson I. Sudden onset headache: a prospective study of features, incidence and causes. Cephalalgia. 2002;22(5): 354–60.
8. Barlow CF. Headaches and migraine in childhood. Clinics in developmental medicine. No. 91. Philadelphia, PA: JB Lippincott; 1984:204–19.
9. Medina LS, Pinter JD, Zurakowski D, Davis RG, Kuban K, Barnes PD. Children with headache: clinical predictors of surgical space-occupying lesions and the role of neuroimaging. Radiology. 1997;202(3):819–24.

10. Weingarten K, Zimmerman RD, Becker RD, Heier LA, Haimes AB, Deck MD. Subdural and epidural empyemas: MR imaging. AJR Am J Roentgenol. 1989;152(3):615–21.
11. Reinus WR, Wippold FJ, Erickson K. Practical selection criteria for unenhanced cranial CT in patients with acute headache. Emerg Radiol. 1994;1:81–4.
12. Reinus WR, Zwemer Jr FL. Clinical prediction of emergent cranial CT results. Ann Emerg Med. 1994;23:1271–8.
13. Reinus WR, Zwemer Jr FL, Wippold FJ, Erickson KK. Emergency imaging of patients with resolved neurologic deficits: value of immediate cranial CT. AJR Am J Roentgenol. 1994;163: 667–70.
14. Aygun D, Bildik F. Clinical warning criteria in evaluation by computed tomography the secondary neurological headaches in adults. Eur J Neurol. 2003;10:437–42.
15. Sobri M, Lamont AC, Alias NA, Win MN. Red flags in patients presenting with headache: clinical indications for neuroimaging. Br J Radiol. 2003;76:532–5.
16. Ramier-Lassepas M, Espinosa C, Cicero JJ, Johnston KL, Clipolle RJ, Barber DL. Predictors of intracranial pathologic findings in patients who see emergency care because of headaches. Arch Neurol. 1997;54:1506–9.
17. Becker L, Iverson DC, Reed FM, Calonge N, Miller RS, Freeman WL. Patients with a new headache in primary care: a report from ASPN. J Fam Pract. 1988;27:41–7.
18. Becker LA, Green LA, Beaufait D, Kirk J, Froom J, Freeman WL. Use of CT scans for the investigation of headache: a report from ASPN, part 1. J Fam Pract. 1993;37:129–34.
19. Morey SS. Headache Consortium releases guidelines for use of CT or MRI in migraine work-up. Am Fam Physician. 2000;62:1699–701.
20. Mettler Jr FA. Essentials of radiology. 2nd ed. Philadelphia, PA: Saunders; 2005.
21. Marx JA, Hockberger RS, Walls JM. Rosen's emergency medicine: concepts and clinical practice. 5th ed. St. Louis, MO: Mosby; 2002.
22. So EL. Classifications and epidemiologic considerations of epileptic seizures and epilepsy. Neuroimaging Clin N Am. 1995;5(4):513–26.
23. Wieshmann UC. Clinical application of neuroimaging in epilepsy. J Neurol Neurosurg Psychiatry. 2003;74(4):466–70.
24. Adams C, Hwang PA, Gilday DL, Armstrong DC, Becker LE, Hoffman HJ. Comparison of SPECT, EEG, CT, MRI, and pathology in partial epilepsy. Pediatr Neurol. 1992;8(2): 97–103.
25. SPECT and PET in epilepsy. Lancet 1989;1(8630):135–7.
26. Bergen D, Bleck T, Ramsey R, et al. Magnetic resonance imaging as a sensitive and specific predictor of neoplasms removed for intractable epilepsy. Epilepsia. 1989;30(3):318–21.
27. Brooks BS, King DW, el Gammal T, et al. MR imaging in patients with intractable complex partial epileptic seizures. AJNR Am J Neuroradiol. 1990;11(1):93–9.
28. Heinz ER, Heinz TR, Radtke R, et al. Efficacy of MR vs CT in epilepsy. AJR Am J Roentgenol. 1989;152(2):347–52.
29. Maxwell RE, Gates JR, McGeachie R. Magnetic resonance imaging in the assessment and surgical management of epilepsy and functional neurological disorders. Appl Neurophysiol. 1987;50(1–6):369–73.
30. Toh KH. Clinical applications of magnetic resonance imaging in the central nervous system. Ann Acad Med Singapore. 1993;22(5):785–93.
31. Cascino GD, Jack Jr CR, Parisi JE, et al. MRI in the presurgical evaluation of patients with frontal lobe epilepsy and children with temporal lobe epilepsy: pathologic correlation and prognostic importance. Epilepsy Res. 1992;11(1):51–9.
32. Jackson GD. New techniques in magnetic resonance and epilepsy. Epilepsia. 1994;35 Suppl 6:S2–13.
33. Spencer SS. The relative contributions of MRI, SPECT, and PET imaging in epilepsy. Epilepsia. 1994;35 Suppl 6:S72–89.
34. Schwartz ES, Dlugos DJ, Storm PB, et al. Magnetoencephalography for pediatric epilepsy: how we do it. AJNR Am J Neuroradiol. 2008;29(5):832–7.

35. Lau M, Yam D, Burneo JG. A systematic review on MEG and its use in the presurgical evaluation of localization-related epilepsy. Epilepsy Res. 2008;79(2–3):97–104.
36. The National Institute of Neurological Disorders and Stroke rt-PA Stroke Study Group. Tissue plasminogen activator for acute ischemic stroke. N Engl J Med. 2010;333:1581–7.
37. Furlan A, Higashida R, Wechsler L, et al. Intra-arterial prourokinase for acute ischemic stroke: The PROACT II study—a randomized controlled trial. Prolyse in acute cerebral thromboembolism. JAMA. 1999;282:2003–11.
38. Kidwell CS, Warach S. Acute ischemic cerebrovascular syndrome: diagnostic criteria. Stroke. 2003;34:2995–8.
39. Easton JD, Saver JL, Albers GW, et al. Definition and evaluation of transient ischemic attack: a scientific statement for healthcare professionals from the American Heart Association/American Stroke Association Stroke Council; Council on Cardiovascular Surgery and Anesthesia; Council on Cardiovascular Radiology and Intervention; Council on Cardiovascular Nursing; and the Interdisciplinary Council on Peripheral Vascular Disease. Stroke. 2009;40:2276–93.
40. Restrepo L, Jacobs MA, Barker PB, Wityk RJ. Assessment of transient ischemic attack with diffusion- and perfusion-weighted imaging. AJNR Am J Neuroradiol. 2004;25:1645–52.
41. Albers GW. Acute cerebrovascular syndrome: time for new terminology for acute brain ischemia. Nat Clin Pract Cardiovasc Med. 2006;3:521.
42. Lloyd-Jones D, Adams R, Carnethon M, et al. Heart disease and stroke statistics—2009 update: a report from the American Heart Association Statistics Committee and Stroke Statistics Subcommittee. Circulation. 2009;119(3):480–6.
43. Rothwell PM, Johnston SC. Transient ischemic attacks: stratifying risk. Stroke. 2006;37(2):320–2.
44. Wintermark M, Meuli R, Browaeys P, et al. Comparison of CT perfusion and angiography and MRI in selecting stroke patients for acute treatment. Neurology. 2007;68(9):694–7.
45. Siebert E, Bohner G, Dewey M, et al. 320-slice CT neuroimaging: initial clinical experience and image quality evaluation. Br J Radiol. 2009;82(979):561–70.
46. Goldstein LB, Adams R, Alberts MJ, et al. Primary prevention of ischemic stroke: a guideline from the American Heart Association/American Stroke Association Stroke Council: cosponsored by the Atherosclerotic Peripheral Vascular Disease Interdisciplinary Working Group; Cardiovascular Nursing Council; Clinical Cardiology Council; Nutrition, Physical Activity, and Metabolism Council; and the Quality of Care and Outcomes Research Interdisciplinary Working Group. Circulation. 2006;113(24):e873–923.
47. Endarterectomy for asymptomatic carotid artery stenosis. Executive Committee for the Asymptomatic Carotid Atherosclerosis Study. JAMA 1995;273(18):1421–8.
48. Barnett HJ, Taylor DW, Eliasziw M, et al. Benefit of carotid endarterectomy in patients with symptomatic moderate or severe stenosis. North American Symptomatic Carotid Endarterectomy Trial Collaborators. N Engl J Med. 1998;339(20):1415–25.
49. Hobson 2nd RW, Weiss DG, Fields WS, et al. Efficacy of carotid endarterectomy for asymptomatic carotid stenosis. The Veterans Affairs Cooperative Study Group. N Engl J Med. 1993;328(4):221–7.
50. Rothwell PM, Eliasziw M, Gutnikov SA, et al. Analysis of pooled data from the randomised controlled trials of endarterectomy for symptomatic carotid stenosis. Lancet. 2003;361(9352):107–16.
51. Brott TG, Hobson 2nd RW, Howard G, et al. Stenting versus endarterectomy for treatment of carotid-artery stenosis. N Engl J Med. 2010;363(1):11–23.
52. Halliday A, Harrison M, Hayter E, et al. 10-year stroke prevention after successful carotid endarterectomy for asymptomatic stenosi (ACST-1): a multicentre randomised trial. Lancet. 2010;376(9746):1074–84.
53. Derdeyn CP, Powers WJ. Cost-effectiveness of screening for asymptomatic carotid atherosclerotic disease. Stroke. 1996;27(11):1944–50.
54. Obuchowski NA, Modic MT, Magdinec M, Masaryk TJ. Assessment of the efficacy of noninvasive screening for patients with asymptomatic neck bruits. Stroke. 1997;28(7):1330–9.

55. Mathiesen EB, Joakimsen O, Bonaa KH. Intersonographer reproducibility and intermethod variability of ultrasound measurements of carotid artery stenosis: The Tromso Study. Cerebrovasc Dis. 2000;10(3):207–13.
56. Wardlaw JM, Chappell FM, Best JJ, Wartolowska K, Berry E. Non-invasive imaging compared with intra-arterial angiography in the diagnosis of symptomatic carotid stenosis: a meta-analysis. Lancet. 2006;367(9521):1503–12.
57. Honish C, Sadanand V, Fladeland D, Chow V, Pirouzmand F. The reliability of ultrasound measurements of carotid stenosis compared to MRA and DSA. Can J Neurol Sci. 2005; 2(4):465–71.
58. Barth A, Arnold M, Mattle HP, Schroth G, Remonda L. Contrastenhanced 3-D MRA in decision making for carotid endarterectomy: a 6-year experience. Cerebrovasc Dis. 2006; 21(5–6):393–400.
59. U-King-Im JM, Hollingworth W, Trivedi RA, et al. Costeffectiveness of diagnostic strategies prior to carotid endarterectomy. Ann Neurol. 2005;58(4):506–15.
60. Bartlett ES, Walters TD, Symons SP, Fox AJ. Quantification of carotid stenosis on CT angiography. AJNR Am J Neuroradiol. 2006;27(1):13–9.
61. Koelemay MJ, Nederkoorn PJ, Reitsma JB, Majoie CB. Systematic review of computed tomographic angiography for assessment of carotid artery disease. Stroke. 2004;35(10): 2306–12.
62. U-King-Im JM, Tang TY, Patterson A, et al. Characterisation of carotid atheroma in symptomatic and asymptomatic patients using high resolution MRI. J Neurol Neurosurg Psychiatry. 2008;79(8):905–12.
63. Wintermark M, Jawadi SS, Rapp JH, et al. High-resolution CT imaging of carotid artery atherosclerotic plaques. AJNR Am J Neuroradiol. 2008;29(5):875–82.
64. Derdeyn CP, Videen TO, Yundt KD, et al. Variability of cerebral blood volume and oxygen extraction: stages of cerebral haemodynamic impairment revisited. Brain. 2002;125 (Pt 3):595–607.
65. Kuroda S, Shiga T, Houkin K, et al. Cerebral oxygen metabolism and neuronal integrity in patients with impaired vasoreactivity attributable to occlusive carotid artery disease. Stroke. 2006;37(2):393–8.
66. Nemoto EM, Yonas H, Kuwabara H, et al. Identification of hemodynamic compromise by cerebrovascular reserve and oxygen extraction fraction in occlusive vascular disease. J Cereb Blood Flow Metab. 2004;24(10):1081–9.
67. Endo H, Inoue T, Ogasawara K, Fukuda T, Kanbara Y, Ogawa A. Quantitative assessment of cerebral hemodynamics using perfusion-weighted MRI in patients with major cerebral artery occlusive disease: comparison with positron emission tomography. Stroke. 2006;37(2): 388–92.
68. Furukawa M, Kashiwagi S, Matsunaga N, Suzuki M, Kishimoto K, Shirao S. Evaluation of cerebral perfusion parameters measured by perfusion CT in chronic cerebral ischemia: comparison with xenon CT. J Comput Assist Tomogr. 2002;26(2):272–8.
69. Adams H, Adams R, Del Zoppo G, Goldstein LB. Guidelines for the early management of patients with ischemic stroke: 2005 guidelines update a scientific statement from the Stroke Council of the American Heart Association/American Stroke Association. Stroke. 2005;36(4):916–23.
70. Hacke W, Donnan G, Fieschi C, et al. Association of outcome with early stroke treatment: pooled analysis of ATLANTIS, ECASS, and NINDS rt-PA stroke trials. Lancet. 2004;363(9411):768–74.
71. Katzan IL, Hammer MD, Furlan AJ, Hixson ED, Nadzam DM. Quality improvement and tissue-type plasminogen activator for acute ischemic stroke: a Cleveland update. Stroke. 2003;34(3):799–800.
72. Reeves MJ, Arora S, Broderick JP, et al. Acute stroke care in the US: results from 4 pilot prototypes of the Paul Coverdell National Acute Stroke Registry. Stroke. 2005;36(6):1232–72.
73. Khatri P, Hill MD, Palesch YY, et al. Methodology of the Interventional Management of Stroke III Trial. Int J Stroke. 2008;3(2):130–7.

74. Mattle HP, Arnold M, Georgiadis D, et al. Comparison of intraarterial and intravenous thrombolysis for ischemic stroke with hyperdense middle cerebral artery sign. Stroke. 2008;39(2):379–83.
75. Smith WS, Sung G, Saver J, et al. Mechanical thrombectomy for acute ischemic stroke: final results of the Multi MERCI trial. Stroke. 2008;39(4):1205–12.
76. De Keyser J, Gdovinova Z, Uyttenboogaart M, Vroomen PC, Luijckx GJ. Intravenous alteplase for stroke: beyond the guidelines and in particular clinical situations. Stroke. 2007;38(9):2612–8.
77. Fiehler J, Albers GW, Boulanger JM, et al. Bleeding risk analysis in stroke imaging before thrombolysis (BRASIL): pooled analysis of T2*-weighted magnetic resonance imaging data from 570 patients. Stroke. 2007;38(10):2738–44.
78. Kohrmann M, Schellinger PD. Acute stroke triage to intravenous thrombolysis and other therapies with advanced CT or MR imaging: pro MR imaging. Radiology. 2009; 251(3):627–33.
79. Adams Jr HP, del Zoppo G, Alberts MJ, et al. Guidelines for the early management of adults with ischemic stroke: a guideline from the American Heart Association/American Stroke Association Stroke Council, Clinical Cardiology Council, Cardiovascular Radiology and Intervention Council, and the Atherosclerotic Peripheral Vascular Disease and Quality of Care Outcomes in Research Interdisciplinary Working Groups: the American Academy of Neurology affirms the value of this guideline as an educational tool for neurologists. Stroke. 2007;38(5):1655–711.
80. Wardlaw JM, Mielke O. Early signs of brain infarction at CT: observer reliability and outcome after thrombolytic treatment—systematic review. Radiology. 2005;235(2):444–53.
81. Wintermark M, Rowley HA, Lev MH. Acute stroke triage to intravenous thrombolysis and other therapies with advanced CT or MR imaging: pro CT. Radiology. 2009;251(3):619–26.
82. Al-Okaili RN, Krejza J, Wang S, Woo JH, Melhem ER. Advanced MR imaging techniques in the diagnosis of intraaxial brain tumors in adults. Radiographics. 2006;26:S173–89.
83. Cross 3rd DT, Tirschwell DL, Clark MA, et al. Mortality rates after subarachnoid hemorrhage: variations according to hospital case volume in 18 states. J Neurosurg. 2003;99(5): 810–7.
84. Flaherty ML, Haverbusch M, Sekar P, et al. Long-term mortality after intracerebral hemorrhage. Neurology. 2006;66(8):1182–6.
85. Black PM. Hydrocephalus and vasospasm after subarachnoid hemorrhage from ruptured intracranial aneurysms. Neurosurgery. 1986;18(1):12–6.
86. Kassell NF, Boarini DJ, Adams Jr HP, et al. Overall management of ruptured aneurysm: comparison of early and late operation. Neurosurgery. 1981;9(2):120–8.
87. Bederson JB, Connolly Jr ES, Batjer HH, et al. Guidelines for the management of aneurysmal subarachnoid hemorrhage: a statement for healthcare professionals from a special writing group of the Stroke Council. American Heart Association. Stroke. 2009;40(3):994–1025.
88. Dammert S, Krings T, Moller-Hartmann W, et al. Detection of intracranial aneurysms with multislice CT: comparison with conventional angiography. Neuroradiology. 2004;46(6):427–34.
89. Jayaraman MV, Mayo-Smith WW, Tung GA, et al. Detection of intracranial aneurysms: multi-detector row CT angiography compared with DSA. Radiology. 2004;230(2):510–8.
90. Li Q, Lv F, Li Y, Luo T, Li K, Xie P. Evaluation of 64-section CT angiography for detection and treatment planning of intracranial aneurysms by using DSA and surgical findings. Radiology. 2009;252(3):808–15.
91. Dehdashti AR, Rufenacht DA, Delavelle J, Reverdin A, de Tribolet N. Therapeutic decision and management of aneurismal subarachnoid haemorrhage based on computed tomographic angiography. Br J Neurosurg. 2003;17(1):46–53.
92. Hoh BL, Cheung AC, Rabinov JD, Pryor JC, Carter BS, Ogilvy CS. Results of a prospective protocol of computed tomographic angiography in place of catheter angiography as the only diagnostic and pretreatment planning study for cerebral aneurysms by a combined neurovascular team. Neurosurgery. 2004;54(6):1329–40; discussion 1340–1322.
93. Aaslid R, Huber P, Nornes H. Evaluation of cerebrovascular spasm with transcranial Doppler ultrasound. J Neurosurg. 1984;60(1):37–41.

94. Kimura T, Shinoda J, Funakoshi T. Prediction of cerebral infarction due to vasospasm following aneurysmal subarachnoid haemorrhage using acetazolamide-activated 123I-IMP SPECT. Acta Neurochir (Wien). 1993;123(3–4):125–8.
95. Kistler JP, Crowell RM, Davis KR, et al. The relation of cerebral vasospasm to the extent and location of subarachnoid blood visualized by CT scan: a prospective study. Neurology. 1983;33(4):424–36.
96. Lewis DH, Eskridge JM, Newell DW, et al. Brain SPECT and the effect of cerebral angioplasty in delayed ischemia due to vasospasm. J Nucl Med. 1992;33(10):1789–96.
97. Sviri GE, Mesiwala AH, Lewis DH, et al. Dynamic perfusion computerized tomography in cerebral vasospasm following aneurysmal subarachnoid hemorrhage: a comparison with technetium-99 m-labeled ethyl cysteinate dimer-single-photon emission computerized tomography. J Neurosurg. 2006;104(3):404–10.
98. Wintermark M, Ko NU, Smith WS, Liu S, Higashida RT, Dillon WP. Vasospasm after subarachnoid hemorrhage: utility of perfusion CT and CT angiography on diagnosis and management. AJNR Am J Neuroradiol. 2006;27(1):26–34.
99. Pouratian N, Oskouian Jr RJ, Jensen ME, Kassell NF, Dumont AS. Endovascular management of unruptured intracranial aneurysms. J Neurol Neurosurg Psychiatry. 2006;77(5):572–8.
100. Wiebers DO, Whisnant JP, Huston 3rd J, et al. Unruptured intracranial aneurysms: natural history, clinical outcome, and risks of surgical and endovascular treatment. Lancet. 2003;362(9378):103–10.
101. Molyneux AJ, Kerr RS, Yu LM, et al. International subarachnoid aneurysm trial (ISAT) of neurosurgical clipping versus endovascular coiling in 2143 patients with ruptured intracranial aneurysms: a randomised comparison of effects on survival, dependency, seizures, rebleeding, subgroups, and aneurysm occlusion. Lancet. 2005;366(9488):809–17.
102. Ruggieri PM, Poulos N, Masaryk TJ, et al. Occult intracranial aneurysms in polycystic kidney disease: screening with MR angiography. Radiology. 1994;191(1):33–9.
103. Ronkainen A, Puranen MI, Hernesniemi JA, et al. Intracranial aneurysms: MR angiographic screening in 400 asymptomatic individuals with increased familial risk. Radiology. 1995;195(1):35–40.
104. Marks MP, Lane B, Steinberg GK, Chang PJ. Hemorrhage in intracerebral arteriovenous malformations: angiographic determinants. Radiology. 1990;176(3):807–13.
105. Spetzler RF, Martin NA. A proposed grading system for arteriovenous malformations. J Neurosurg. 1986;65(4):476–83.
106. Cronqvist M, Wirestam R, Ramgren B, et al. Endovascular treatment of intracerebral arteriovenous malformations: procedural safety, complications, and results evaluated by MR imaging, including diffusion and perfusion imaging. AJNR Am J Neuroradiol. 2006;27(1):162–76.
107. Gupta V, Chugh M, Walia BS, Vaishya S, Jha AN. Use of CT angiography for anatomic localization of arteriovenous malformation Nidal components. AJNR Am J Neuroradiol. 2008;29(10):1837–40.
108. Lanzino G, Fraser K, Kanaan Y, Wagenbach A. Treatment of ruptured intracranial aneurysms since the International Subarachnoid Aneurysm Trial: practice utilizing clip ligation and coil embolization as individual or complementary therapies. J Neurosurg. 2006;104(3):344–9.
109. Molyneux AJ, Kerr RS, Yu LM, et al. International subarachnoid aneurysm trial (ISAT) of neurosurgical clipping versus endovascular coiling in 2143 patients with ruptured intracranial aneurysms: a randomised comparison of effects on survival, dependency, seizures, rebleeding, subgroups, and aneurysm occlusion. Lancet. 2005;36(9488):809–17.
110. Schaafsma JD, Koffijberg H, Buskens E, Velthuis BK, van der Graaf Y, Rinkel GJ. Cost-effectiveness of magnetic resonance angiography versus intra-arterial digital subtraction angiography to follow-up patients with coiled intracranial aneurysms. Stroke. 2010;41(8):1736–42.
111. Sprengers ME, Schaafsma JD, van Rooij WJ, et al. Evaluation of the occlusion status of coiled intracranial aneurysms with MR angiography at 3 T: is contrast enhancement necessary? AJNR Am J Neuroradiol. 2009;30(9):1665–71.
112. Shellock FG, Crues JV. MR procedures: biologic effects, safety, and patient care. Radiology. 2004;232(3):635–52.

Chapter 3
Cardiothoracic Imaging

Robert M. Steiner, Chandra A. Dass, and Scott A. Simpson

Introduction

Diseases that involve the heart, lungs, pleura, and mediastinum present with a variety of acute signs and symptoms. A number of imaging technologies are integral to the diagnosis and management of acute thoracic disease. Some, such as the chest radiograph, are as old as the field of radiology itself. Others, such as nuclear imaging and ultrasonography, are more recent in development, but today are considered mature modalities. Still others, including computed tomography (CT) and magnetic resonance imaging (MRI), have grown in importance in recent years because the quality of images from these modalities has improved markedly. As a result the number of applications to which they are applied also has expanded greatly, in some cases displacing other imaging modalities as the first line modality. Regardless, each imaging modality has unique advantages, limitations, and indications resulting in development of increasingly complex clinical algorithms for their appropriate application. Furthermore, the relative cost, potential complications, and radiation dose of each of these modalities impact their utilization.

Chest Radiography

The standard two-view erect radiographic study of the chest is typically the starting point for evaluation of thoracic pathology. This study includes both posterior-anterior (PA) and lateral (LAT) projections. Other specialized views, including apical lordotic, decubitus, and oblique projections, are used occasionally. For example, the apical lordotic projection better visualizes the lung apices than a standard PA

R.M. Steiner, M.D. (✉) • C.A. Dass, M.D. • S.A. Simpson, M.D.
Department of Radiology, Temple University Hospital, Philadelphia, PA 19140, USA
e-mail: rsteiner5933@aol.com

W.R. Reinus (ed.), *Clinician's Guide to Diagnostic Imaging*,
DOI 10.1007/978-1-4614-8769-2_3, © Springer Science+Business Media New York 2014

view, and lateral decubitus views show whether fluid in the pleural space is loculated or free-flowing.

When a patient is too ill to be positioned for a standard two-view chest study, a portable chest study (PCR) in the anteroposterior (AP) projection may be obtained instead. Portable radiographs generally are poorer in quality than standard two-view examinations because the X-ray generators used on portable machines are less powerful than standard stationary generators; patients may not be able to suspend respiration for the duration of the exposure and patient positioning for the study is not standardized. This means that the PCR may not show either anatomy or pathology in a reproducible fashion. Obtaining diagnostic studies of unstable or uncooperative patients and in those who have numerous life support lines and catheters also presents unique challenges that lead to reduced diagnostic quality [1]. Nevertheless, this technique is used frequently in the care of acutely ill or immobilized patients.

Computed Tomography

CT uses X-ray to create cross-sectional images. Volumetric CT, the current state of the art, is performed by moving the patient through the machine's gantry at a constant speed as imaging data is acquired usually within a single breath-hold [2, 3]. This technique is known as multidetector computed tomography (MDCT) and has enabled rapid image acquisition of large volumes of tissue. This means that CT can reimage a patient in different vascular phases after a single intravenous contrast bolus. Although MDCT has broadened the indications for CT, it also has led to a dramatic increase in radiation dose on a per study basis, not just for thoracic indications but for all body organ systems. Increased radiation raises concern for increased risk of cancer induction years after the CT study and is especially concerning in younger more radiosensitive patients and in those patients studied as part of screening protocols [4, 5].

Indications for thoracic CT can be broadly divided into clinical scenarios where more detail is needed to clarify a finding suggested on other imaging modalities, such as plain radiographs or radionuclide studies, and those in which thoracic disease is suspected on clinical grounds alone [6] (Table 3.1).

Radionuclide Imaging

Ventilation/perfusion (V/Q) scans are designed to diagnose pulmonary embolism (PE) and are the most commonly obtained nuclear study of the lungs [7, 8]. It involves simultaneous imaging of pulmonary blood flow and alveolar ventilation. According to a recent American College of Radiology Appropriateness Criteria Committee report, these scans are particularly sensitive for the diagnosis of chronic pulmonary thromboembolic disease. Today, they are also used to diagnose acute PE in patients who cannot undergo a contrast CT.

Table 3.1 Clinical indications for thoracic CT

Abnormal chest X-ray
- Workup of patient with suspected COPD for consideration for lung volume reduction or transplant
- Assessment of possible aortic dissection, aneurysm, or aortic ulcer
- Characterization of diffuse lung disease

Chest X-ray is normal or noncontributary
- Identification of unrecognized lung disease in symptomatic patients
- Detection of metastatic disease or a suspected solitary pulmonary nodule
- Demonstration of pulmonary embolism
- Visualization of aortic dissection
- Investigation of the patient with fever, hemoptysis, shortness of breath, or wheezing
- Clinical disease likely to be thoracic in etiology, e.g., myasthenia gravis, carcinoid syndrome, or paraneoplastic syndromes

Magnetic Resonance Imaging

Imaging with MR presents unique challenges because of the low inherent MR signal intensity of lung and the deleterious effects of respiratory and cardiac motion on MR image acquisition. The tissue-air interfaces in lungs cause image distorting artifacts and loss of coherent signal. Motion artifact and image ghosting are more evident in studies performed on high field strength imagers compared with lower field strength magnets. Although careful manipulation of technical factors such as cardiac and respiratory gating can improve image quality, pulmonary MR remains difficult to achieve and for this reason indications for pulmonary MR remain limited [9]. Nonetheless, because MRI has excellent soft tissue resolution, it is useful for identification of tumor invasion into the chest wall and mediastinum. It is also useful to differentiate solid from cystic masses and to demonstrate diaphragmatic abnormalities [10].

MRI along with magnetic resonance angiography (MRA) has been shown to be highly accurate for the diagnosis of thoracic aortic disease, with sensitivities and specificities that are equivalent to those for MDCT and transesophageal echocardiography (TEE). Velocity-encoded phase contrast flow quantification techniques enable measurement of the differential flow velocity in the true and false channels and evaluation of aortic valve motion. Since no radiation is involved, MRI may be preferred over MDCT for patients who require repeated imaging. MRI is also useful to diagnose various causes of chest pain and may be helpful to characterize both ischemic and non-ischemic cardiomyopathies such as hypertrophic and dilated cardiomyopathy. Infiltrative cardiomyopathy due to sarcoidosis, amyloidosis, or tumor among other conditions may be characterized by MRI (Table 3.2).

Table 3.2 Clinical indications for thoracic MRI

• *Aorta*: Aortic dissection, aneurysm, aortitis, coarctation, cardiac valvular flow and function
• *Pulmonary arteries*: Pulmonary embolism, vasculitis, pulmonary hypertension
• *Lung*: Pancoast tumors, neoplastic chest wall invasion
• *Heart*: Myocardial and pericardial disease
• *Mediastinum*: Identification and characterization of neoplasm

Angiography

In recent years, there has been a shift in the imaging strategy for diseases of the aorta from invasive catheter aortography to noninvasive approaches. MDCT angiography (CTA), echocardiography and MRI are currently the first line imaging tests for the diagnostic work-up of thoracic aortic pathology.

CT arteriography (CTA) is the most commonly requested diagnostic test for suspected acute or chronic thoracic aortic disease. Because aortic disease is commonly diffuse or multifocal, the scanning field typically extends from thoracic inlet to the aortic bifurcation. The imaging field may be extended further to involve the proximal femoral vessels, if intervention is contemplated. A non-enhanced scan is usually performed first to look for (a) high-attenuation acute intramural hematoma, (b) distribution of calcification, and (c) as a baseline to access enhancement of the aortic wall and para-aortic tissue. After rapid IV injection of iodinated contrast for the CTA portion of the study, images are acquired during patient "breath holding" to reduce respiratory artifacts. Electrocardiographic (ECG) gating is commonly used to reduce cardiac motion artifacts, particularly when evaluating the ascending aorta. In addition, ECG gating can facilitate visualization of the proximal coronary arteries. Electrocardiographic gating is turned off at the diaphragm to reduce both breath-hold time and radiation dose. Two dimensional (2D) and three dimensional (3D) reformatting techniques, such as multiplanar reconstruction (MPR), maximum intensity projection (MIP), volume rendering (VR), and direct endoluminal viewing, are used according to the clinical indications for the study (Table 3.3).

Echocardiography

The primary role of transthoracic echocardiography (TTE) is to image the aortic root and ascending aorta. It does not consistently visualize the mid or distal ascending or the descending aorta. TEE has higher sensitivity and specificity than TTE [11]. TEE can visualize more of the aorta wall than TTE, but it may not visualize the distal ascending aorta, proximal arch, and the proximal abdominal aorta. TEE can be performed both at the bedside with the patient under sedation and

Table 3.3 Advantages and disadvantages of CT angiography

Advantages
1. Easy availability, most often within or near the emergency department
2. Short imaging time, easy patient monitoring while scanning
3. Ability to image the entire aorta and its branches as well as organ perfusion
4. Ability to study the aortic wall, and periaortic tissues
5. Evaluate the rest of the chest and abdomen for a possible alternative diagnosis
Disadvantages
1. Motion artifact may mimic aortic pathology
2. Image degradation by implanted devices, catheters, and leads
3. Exposure to ionizing radiation and IV iodinated contrast

intraoperatively. Ultrasound does not expose the patient to radiation and no injection of contrast material is necessary. Beyond establishing the presence of aortic pathology, echocardiography can also be used to evaluate concomitant cardiac disease. Given the semi-invasive nature of TEE, MDCT scan is favored for the routine imaging of stable patients.

Clinical Scenarios

Shortness of Breath

Shortness of breath (dyspnea), whether acute or chronic, most often is either pulmonary or cardiovascular in etiology. Frequent cardiovascular causes of dyspnea include acute coronary syndrome (ACS), congestive heart failure, and a variety of cardiomyopathies. Pulmonary etiologies include chronic obstructive pulmonary disease (asthma, emphysema, and chronic bronchitis), pulmonary hypertension, pneumothorax, PE, airway obstruction, and interstitial lung disease [12]. Distinguishing clinically between cardiovascular and pulmonary etiologies can be difficult. At times, disease involving both systems may contribute to a patient's shortness of breath.

Chest radiography and ECG are usually the initial studies of choice in the workup of a patient with acute shortness of breath [13]. The results of these studies can help to direct further workup. MDCT is currently the best imaging tool to assess diffuse lung disease, especially when clinical evaluation and laboratory studies as well as plain film radiographs are non-diagnostic [14, 15]. In some cases performing the study prone and/or in the expiratory phase may be helpful to evaluate the pattern of air trapping. Many conditions such as bronchiectasis, emphysema, sarcoidosis, and lymphangetic spread of neoplasm have characteristic imaging features on MDCT that permit a specific diagnosis or at least a limited differential, even when the chest radiograph is normal [16]. Computed tomography is the most sensitive technique for the identification of emphysema in cigarette smokers and can provide unique phenotypic information in COPD [17].

Contrast enhancement is useful to assess many cases of acute dyspnea because it can help to identify vascular etiologies such as PE, aortic dissection, and coronary artery disease. ECG gating is essential for the evaluation of both dissection and coronary artery disease because cardiac motion causes artifacts that limit the diagnostic capabilities of CT.

Pneumothorax

Pneumothorax is defined as collapse of all or part of a lung replaced by air in the pleural space. Pneumothorax may be primary without an identifiable cause or secondary to an iatrogenic procedure, trauma, or underlying lung disorders such as interstitial lung disease or emphysema. Since the advent of CT, most primary pneumothoraces have been shown to arise from rupture of small apical blebs that are not apparent on chest radiographs. A tension pneumothorax, because of the increased pressure in the pleural space on the side of the pneumothorax, causes mass effect on the cardiomediastinum and displaces it toward the contralateral hemithorax.

Because of lower cost, radiation, and ready availability, a chest radiograph is most commonly used to diagnose a suspected pneumothorax (Fig. 3.1). The sensitivity of radiographs for the detection of pneumothoraces is greatly influenced by patient positioning. Whenever possible, an upright PA view of the chest should be performed. This allows air not contained by loculations to track superiorly toward the lung apex such that the classic appearance of a visceral pleural line can be detected. If the radiograph fails to show the pneumothorax, a lateral decubitus (affected side up) or upright expiratory views can be acquired. It should be noted that the use of expiratory radiographs is controversial and when used alone can limit chest X-ray interpretation by creating false linear opacities. CT is the gold standard for the diagnosis of a pneumothorax with near 100 % sensitivity, but it gives a higher dose of radiation, costs more, and is not as available as radiography.

Unstable patients or those debilitated by trauma may not be able to tolerate a standard PA chest radiograph. In these cases a portable AP view of the chest may be performed at the bedside [18]. Should the patient remain in a fully upright position, little is lost in terms of sensitivity. The sensitivity for detection of pneumothorax on supine or semi-recumbent films decreases to around 28 % compared with 92 % on a fully upright PA view of the chest. This is the consequence of air tracking to the anteromedial pleural space when a patient is recumbent.

An occult pneumothorax is one that is not seen on conventional radiographs and only detectable on more advanced imaging. By comparing CT with supine AP radiographs in patients who have had trauma, the incidence of occult pneumothorax has been calculated to average approximately 5 %. The incidence varied considerably, ranging from 4 % in injured children, 22 and 17 % percent in blunt and penetrating trauma, and 64 % in multi-trauma intubated patients [19, 20].

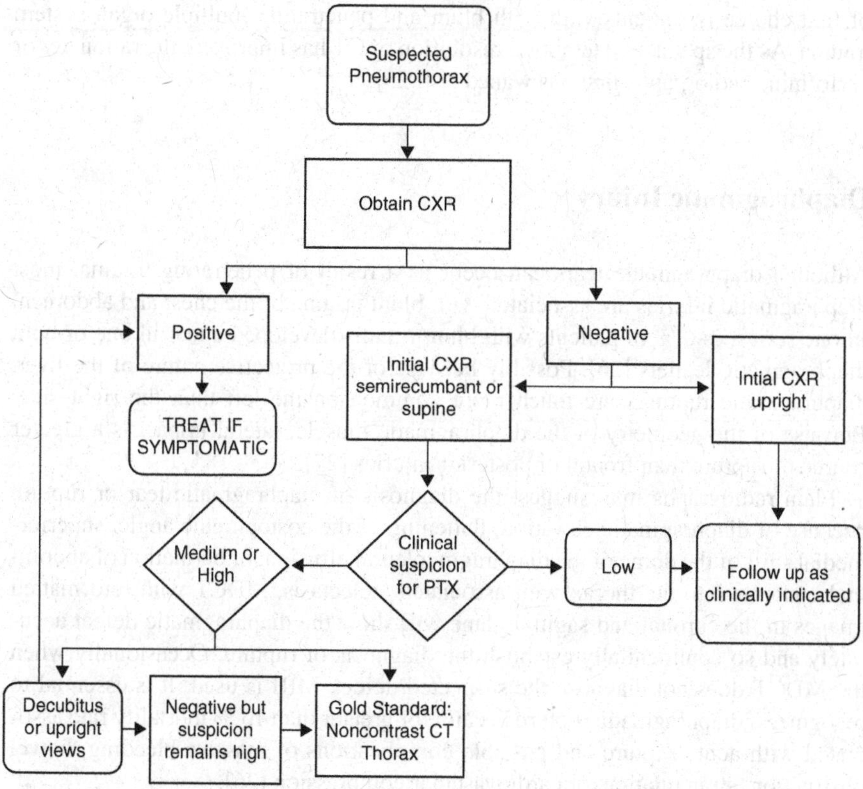

Fig. 3.1 Evaluation of pneumothorax

Thoracic Trauma

After head and musculoskeletal injuries, thoracic trauma is the leading cause of morbidity and mortality, particularly in younger individuals. In a series of 24,000 patients with multiple injuries at a Level 1 trauma center, 70 % included CNS injuries, 90 % musculoskeletal injuries, and over 50 % thoracic injuries [21]. The major causes of thoracic trauma include blunt trauma typically related to a fall, crush injury, explosion, or most commonly a motor vehicle accident. In 2001, for example, 45 % of blunt traumatic injuries were related to MVA [22]. Penetrating trauma is usually caused by knife or bullet injuries. These cause focal lung and soft tissue damage such as laceration, pneumothorax, pneumatocoele, pulmonary contusion, tracheobronchial, vascular, cardiac, and pericardial injury [23].

The plain chest radiograph is usually the first study performed for thoracic trauma. Since the plain chest X-ray is usually performed in the recumbent position, life -threatening injuries such as cardiac bruise and aortic rupture leading to pseudoaneurysm may be difficult to identify. For these reasons CT has become the study of first choice in patients with both blunt and penetrating multiple organ system trauma. As the spatial and temporal resolution of CT has improved, the rationale for performing radiographs first has waned [24, 25].

Diaphragmatic Injury

Although diaphragmatic tears can occur as a result of penetrating trauma, most diaphragmatic injuries are associated with blunt trauma of the chest and abdomen. In one series, 3–6 % of patients with blunt trauma developed a tear in one or both diaphragmatic leaflets [26]. Possibly because of the protective nature of the liver, diaphragmatic ruptures are much more common on the left than the right side. Because of the geometry of the diaphragmatic muscle, lateral impact is a greater source of rupture than frontal or posterior injuries [27].

Plain radiographs may suggest the diagnosis of diaphragmatic tear or rupture because of diaphragmatic elevation, flattening of the costophrenic angle, superior-medial shift of the dome of the diaphragm, pleural effusion, or herniation of abdominal contents into the thorax with associated atelectasis. MDCT with reformatted images in the coronal and sagittal plane will show the diaphragmatic defect accurately and so confidentially establish the diagnosis of rupture. Occasionally when the MDCT does not diagnose the suspected defect, MRI is used. It is essential to recognize a diaphragmatic rupture because of greater than 15 % mortality rate associated with acute rupture and possible complications of massive bleeding, bowel obstruction, strangulation, or cardiovascular compression [26].

Sternal Injury

Sternal fractures occur in up to 4 % of patients with severe blunt trauma. They most often occur near or at the angle of Louis and may be associated with a retrosternal hematoma. Because of the orientation of the fracture it will be best demonstrated with a lateral chest X-ray or by CT. Sternal fractures may be associated with anterior rib fractures, cardiac contusion, pericardial herniation, hemopericardium, and aortic or other vascular injury [28].

Tracheobronchial Rupture

Tracheobronchial injury can occur in up to 3 % of patients from sudden tissue compression related to high velocity blunt trauma, such as a steering wheel injury. The usual sites of rupture are the main stem bronchi in 90 % and the distal trachea in 10 % of patients. Findings that suggest the diagnosis of bronchial rupture include pneumomediastinum, tension pneumothorax, and subcutaneous emphysema. Deformity of the involved airway and downward displacement of the detached lung, also termed the "Falling Lung Sign," are strong clues to the diagnosis. Although the diagnosis of tracheobronchial rupture can occasionally be made on plain radiographs, MDCT is preferred since the tracheobronchial tree can be reconstructed in multiple planes and CT is more sensitive to detect ancillary findings [29, 30].

Acute Thoracic Aortic Injury

The majority of cases of acute aortic injury occur in patients with multisystem trauma, most often motor vehicle accidents. Nearly, 80–90 % of all patients with aortic laceration have a complete tear through the wall of the aorta and exsanguinate and die at the scene of the accident or at the hospital before initiation of treatment [30]. Patients who survive to be imaged often have partial aortic tears with intact adventitia, resulting in a contained rupture or minimal aortic injury affecting only the intimal layer of the aorta [30].

The vast majority of traumatic aortic tears occur at the aortic isthmus, within 2 cm. of the origin of the left subclavian artery. Traumatic injuries to the ascending aorta have a high acute mortality rate and so are uncommonly seen on imaging. These usually occur just distal to the aortic valve and often coexist with myocardial contusion, aortic valve rupture, and/or hemopericardium. Traumatic involvement of aortic arch and branch vessels is also less common, but potentially fatal. The extent of branch vessel injuries, like aortic injuries, ranges from subtle intimal injuries to complete transection and contained rupture. Mid and distal descending thoracic aortic involvement is uncommon, often occurring near the diaphragmatic hiatus.

A portable supine chest radiograph should be obtained initially to identify life-threatening lesions requiring immediate intervention, e.g., massive hemothorax or tension pneumothorax (Fig. 3.2). Another reason to obtain a chest radiograph is to diagnose a mediastinal hematoma, which may suggest a significant vascular injury. A widened mediastinum is the most common finding associated with mediastinal hematoma, others include blurring of the aortic outline, loss of the aortopulmonary window, left apical pleural cap, and right tracheal deviation. Unfortunately, a widened mediastinum on a portable chest radiograph is neither sensitive nor specific for acute aortic injury. Thus, a more definitive diagnostic test should be performed, regardless of the chest radiographic findings.

MDCT/CTA is currently the diagnostic test of choice for the definitive evaluation of acute aortic injury. The imaging protocol is similar to that for aortic dissection. Aortic injury is diagnosed using both direct and indirect signs. The most common indirect finding is a mediastinal hematoma. Periaortic hematoma that is contiguous with the aortic wall is an indeterminate finding for the source of bleeding and so the possibility of an aortic tear should be investigated further. Direct signs of aortic injury include intimal flap, pseudoaneurysm, focal contour abnormality, intramural hematoma, mural thrombus, and abrupt change in luminal caliber

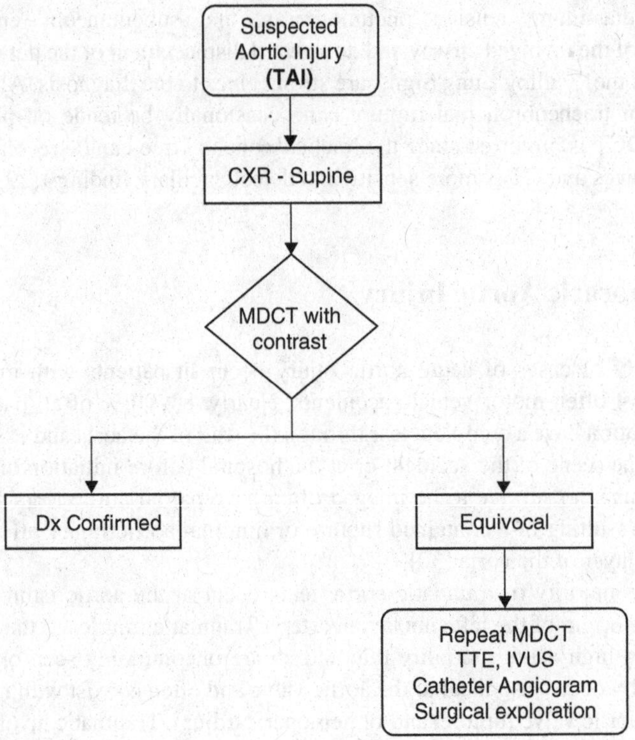

Fig. 3.2 Aortic Trauma Schematic

(pseudocoarctation). Direct findings are usually definitive, and unless there are extenuating circumstances, no additional imaging is necessary. If the aortic adventitia is breached, frank active extravasation of contrast from the aortic lumen is seen, but this is a rare imaging finding and often portends impending exsanguination.

Minimal aortic injuries, e.g., intimal flaps, are better visualized using high-resolution diagnostic techniques and multidetector scanners. In contrast to more severe aortic injury, in-hospital mortality from minimal aortic injury usually is not related to the aortic injury itself, and so these injuries may be amenable to conservative management. Nevertheless, close imaging surveillance to detect an adverse course of a minimal aortic injury is mandatory [31].

Acutely, MRI has a limited role in trauma patients because of logistical issues. MRI and MRA may have value once patients are stable when surgery is contemplated and minimal or equivocal intimal injuries are present. Of course, MRI eliminates the problem of radiation exposure in younger trauma victims [32].

When both MDCT and intra-arterial aortographic studies are inconclusive, intravascular ultrasonography (IVUS) can be helpful to diagnose traumatic aortic injury. It is invasive, requiring arterial puncture, and thus is ideally performed concurrently in association with catheter aortography. IVUS is an operator- and experience-dependent modality, and complete evaluation of the aorta can be time-consuming.

TEE is another modality that can be employed to evaluate the aorta when MDCT/CTA or intra-arterial aortographic studies are equivocal. TEE is widely available, minimally invasive, and can be performed quickly at the bedside or in the operating room. Since TEE is performed in real-time, the aortic valve, sinotubular junction, and ascending aorta can be evaluated to a much better extent with TEE than with MDCT [33].

Pericardial and Cardiac Trauma

Injury to the heart and/or the pericardium occurs in more than 2 % of serious chest trauma following a motor vehicle accident resulting from high energy impact followed by rapid deceleration [34]. Pneumohemopericardium, cardiac herniation, myocardial contusion, valve leaflet tear, aortic rupture, and ventricular septal defect have been described. While radiographs may show a sudden change in the size of the cardiac silhouette, CT with intravenous contrast is the preferred modality for diagnosis when pericardial or cardiac CT is suspected.

Imaging the Patient with Fever

While there are many causes of fever in the acute setting, pulmonary etiologies are particularly common. Viral, bacterial, and fungal infections, tuberculosis, tumor and noninfectious inflammatory conditions such as collagen-vascular disease, medications and illicit drugs such as cocaine, and heat exhaustion are among the many sources of respiratory-induced fever.

The role of the radiologist is to confirm the presence of an acute pulmonary abnormality and, if possible, narrow the differential diagnosis. Typically, plain radiographs suffice for this purpose. Lateral decubitus films may be helpful when pleural fluid is suspected but not confirmed by the PA and lateral projections. Decubitus views are especially important when an erect frontal and lateral examination cannot be performed. If the pneumonia is refractory to treatment or is suspected to be secondary to another source of pathology, e.g., neoplasm obstructing a bronchus, a CT scan of the thorax may be of value. CT scanning is also useful when a cavity is identified and a mycetoma is suspected. Furthermore, CT is useful in the diagnosis and staging of empyema, septic emboli, and fistulous tracts as one might see in actinomycosis or tuberculosis. Otherwise, the majority of pneumonias can be diagnosed and followed using standard radiographs. The frequency of and requirement for the performance of follow-up chest radiographs depend on the patient's clinical status. In routine cases if the patient is recovering with cessation of fever and respiratory complaints, no further films are needed. On the other hand, some patents such as those with altered immune status should be followed at least monthly until the infiltrate has resolved [32].

Imaging the Patient with Hemoptysis

Although in most cases true hemoptysis, that is blood originating from the tracheobronchial tree and not the nasopharynx or GI tract, is not massive or life-threatening, it may be the harbinger of significant pathology. Common causes of hemoptysis include bronchitis (29 %), bronchogenic carcinoma (<29 %), bronchiectasis (25 % of patients), pneumonia (<20 %), pulmonary emboli (10 %), CHF (5 %), and vasculitis (<5 %) [35].

Controversy exists over the most efficacious diagnostic pathway to identify the etiology of hemoptysis. If a chest radiograph is unrevealing, both bronchoscopy and CT have been considered the next procedure of choice. On the one hand, bronchoscopy not only can provide direct visualization of the cause of the hemoptysis, but it also permits biopsy at the time of the procedure. If the bleeding is substantial, however, the airways may be filled with blood making bronchoscopic evaluation of the distal airways difficult. CT is noninvasive and is more likely than bronchoscopy to detect the underlying etiology of the bleeding [34]. In a study of 80 patients with large amounts of hemoptysis by Revel et al., the chest X-ray was normal in 13 %, revealed the cause of bleeding in 35 % and the site of bleeding in 46 %. CT was more efficient than bronchoscopy at identifying the etiology of the bleeding (77 % vs. 8 %) whereas the two modalities were comparable in identifying the site of bleeding [34]. The authors suggested that chest CT should replace bronchoscopy as the first line procedure for the evaluation of large amounts of hemoptysis.

The Solitary Pulmonary Nodule

The most important clinical question regarding a solitary pulmonary nodule (SPN) is whether or not it represents a malignancy [36]. An SPN is an opacity of less than 3 cm in diameter surrounded by normal lung parenchyma without associated atelectasis, pleural effusions, or adenopathy on chest radiography. Often, an SPN is discovered incidentally on radiographs obtained for other reasons. Because CT has better resolution than chest X-ray, an SPN can be characterized with CT as solid, mixed, semisolid, or ground glass. The presence of calcification and cavitation may also be seen to advantage with CT (Fig. 3.3).

Only two imaging features of an SPN clearly exclude malignancy: a benign calcification pattern within the nodule and a solid lesion that is stable over a 2-year period. A ground glass or mixed lesion may represent adenocarcinoma in situ or bronchioalveolar carcinoma, which may show imaging stability for 2 years but then occasionally may exhibit later growth. Since other characteristics such as irregular borders, cavitation and shape do not exclude or definitively characterize an SPN as malignant, most lesions remain indeterminate.

Lesion size is a valuable indicator or possible malignancy. An SPN larger than 1 cm in diameter is much more likely to be malignant than a smaller nodule. A lesion of 6 mm is 30 times more likely to be benign than one that is larger [35].

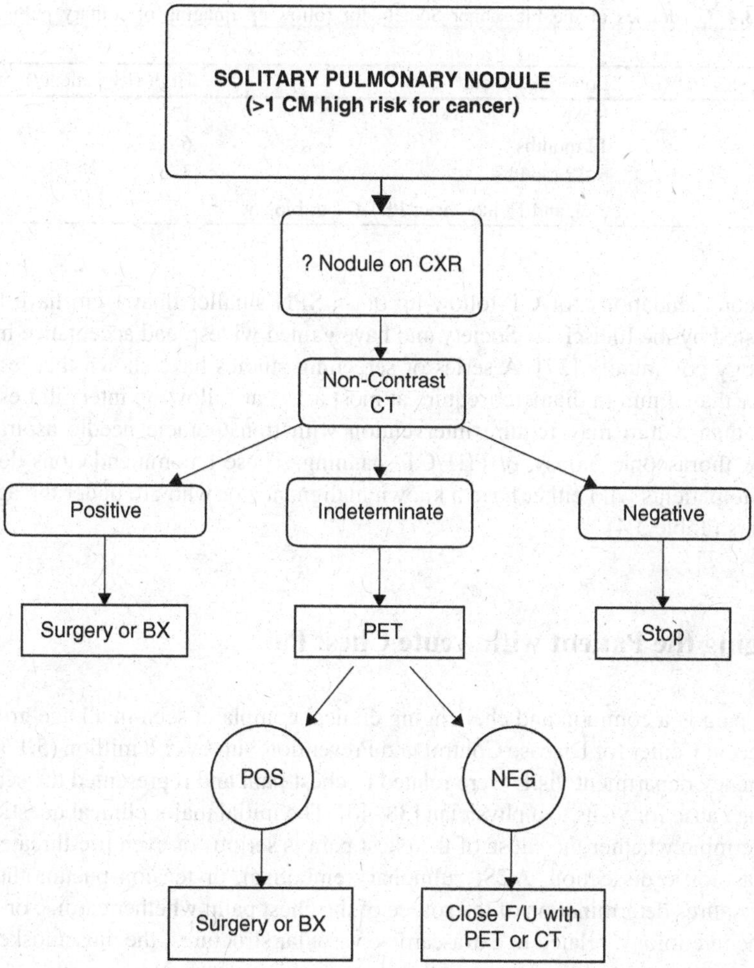

Fig. 3.3 Evaluation of the solitary pulmonary nodule

The rate of growth of an SPN is also important. The typical lung cancer will double in volume in 4.2–7.3 months depending on cell type. A few will take up to 24 months and a few will double in as little as 1 month. Doubling times of less than 1 month suggest inflammatory disease, aggressive lymphoma, or aggressive metastases. Doubling times greater than 18 months suggest granuloma, carcinoid, hamartoma, or rounded atelectasis.

Positron emission tomography (PET) combined with CT has been used mainly in lesions larger than 7 mm in diameter. PET/CT may suggest malignancy when the FDG levels are elevated sufficiently. Certain types of adenocarcinoma and typical carcinoids have low FDG levels and may be confused with benign disease. An inflammatory SPN may have elevated FDG and be confused with low-grade malignant lesions. Thus, PET/CT is useful but not foolproof for the diagnosis of malignant versus benign SPN.

Table 3.4 Guidelines of the Fleischner Society for follow-up imaging of solitary pulmonary nodules

Nodule size (mm)	Low-risk patient	High-risk patient (months)
<4	None	12
4–6	12 months	6–12
6–8	6–12 months	3–6
>8	3, 6, and 12 months or PET/CT or biopsy	

Recommendations for CT follow-up of an SPN smaller than 1 cm have been suggested by the Fleischner Society and have gained widespread acceptance in the radiology community [37]. A series of screening studies have shown that lesions smaller than 4 mm in diameter require at most a 1 year follow-up interval. Lesions larger than 8 mm may require intervention with transthoracic needle aspiration biopsy, thoracoscopic biopsy, or PET/CT scanning. These recommendations do not apply to patients who either have a known malignancy or who are under the age of 35 years (Table 3.4).

Imaging the Patient with Acute Chest Pain

Chest pain is a common and challenging clinical complaint seen in all age groups. In a recent Center for Disease Control and Prevention Survey, 5.8 million (5.1 %) of emergency department visits were related to chest pain and represented the second leading cause for visits to a physician [38–40]. The initial major clinical question is to determine whether the cause of the chest pain is serious or even life-threatening such as aortic dissection, ACS, pulmonary embolism, or tension pneumothorax. This requires determination of the source of the chest pain: whether cardiac or non-cardiac in etiology, related to extra-cardiac vascular structures, the musculoskeletal system, the gastrointestinal tract, or the lungs.

Task forces of the American College of Chest Physicians and the American College of Radiology have addressed the problem of diagnosing the etiology of acute chest pain. They suggest the use of ECG and serum cardiac markers as the first diagnostic measures. When appropriate, these are followed by chest radiography – to exclude pneumothorax or pulmonary edema. Echocardiography, V/Q scan, resting nuclear perfusion scanning, and CTA should be used to exclude pulmonary embolism and aortic dissection [41, 42]. More recently, CT coronary angiography has become a major imaging modality to establish the presence or absence of occlusive cardiovascular disease in patients with acute chest pain [43].

Incorrect triaging of patients with serious acute pain is a common problem. In a study of over 10,000 patients with chest pain and other symptoms, 2.3 % of patients with unstable angina and 2.1 % of those patients who were later shown to have an acute myocardial infarction were discharged from the hospital inappropriately. In addition, many patients were admitted to the hospital for further investigation who

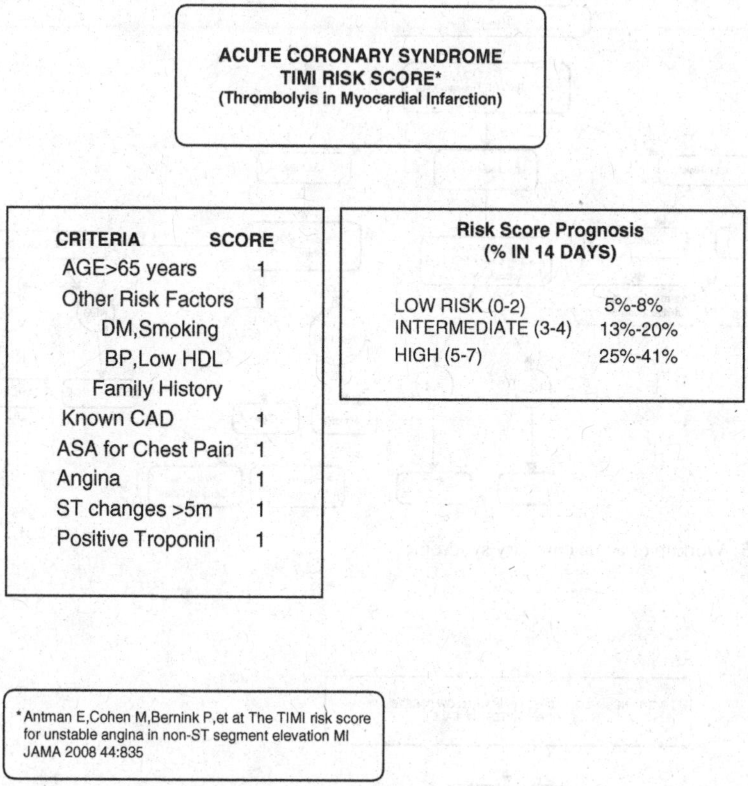
ACUTE CORONARY SYNDROME
TIMI RISK SCORE*
(Thrombolyis in Myocardial Infarction)
CRITERIA SCORE
AGE>65 years 1
Other Risk Factors 1
DM,Smoking
BP,Low HDL
Family History
Known CAD 1
ASA for Chest Pain 1
Angina 1
ST changes >5m 1
Positive Troponin 1
Risk Score Prognosis
(% IN 14 DAYS)
LOW RISK (0-2) 5%-8%
INTERMEDIATE (3-4) 13%-20%
HIGH (5-7) 25%-41%
*Antman E,Cohen M,Bernink P,et at The TIMI risk score
for unstable angina in non-ST segment elevation MI
JAMA 2008 44:835

Fig. 3.4 TIMI risk triaging for acute coronary syndrome

proved not to have serious sources of chest pain and could have been discharged from the emergency department [44].

Patients with chest pain may be divided into three groups (Fig. 3.4). The first has clear evidence of an ACS based on physical examination, ECG findings, and a positive biomarker determination (Fig. 3.5). These patients will be admitted to the hospital for cardiac angiography and intervention procedures. The second category includes patients whose symptoms are less serious and in most cases these patients are discharged with symptomatic medication. The third group includes patients where the clinical profile is less clear cut. They are usually middle-aged individuals with chest pain that is not clearly cardiac in origin and ECG and laboratory values that are equivocal (Figs. 3.6 and 3.7). Unfortunately, this last group comprises a significant proportion of patients presenting with acute chest pain. In these patients, noninvasive diagnostic imaging such as CT coronary angiography has an important role in separating those patients with serious cardiac disease from those with chest pain of other etiologies. Occasionally, radionuclide perfusion imaging, echocardiography and, in selected cases, MR are helpful.

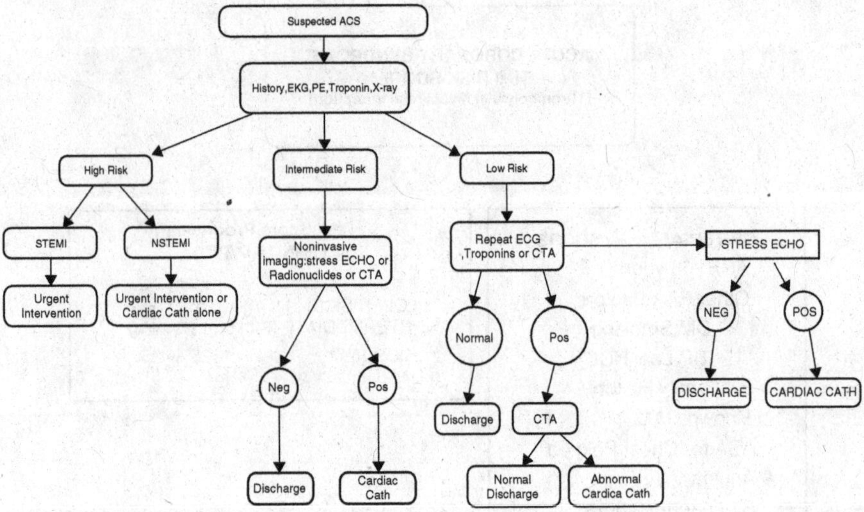

Fig. 3.5 Workup of acute coronary syndrome

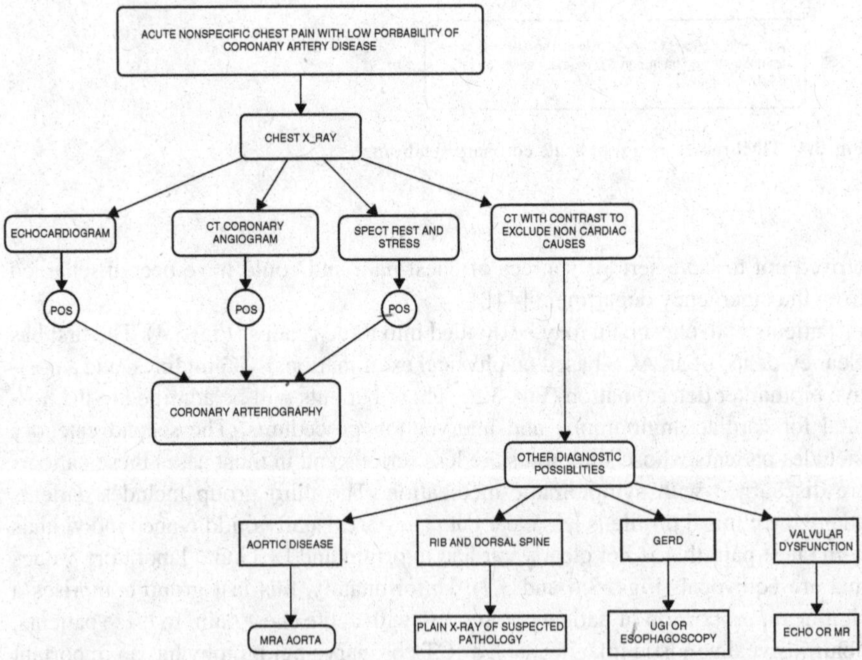

Fig. 3.6 Evaluation of nonspecific acute chest pain

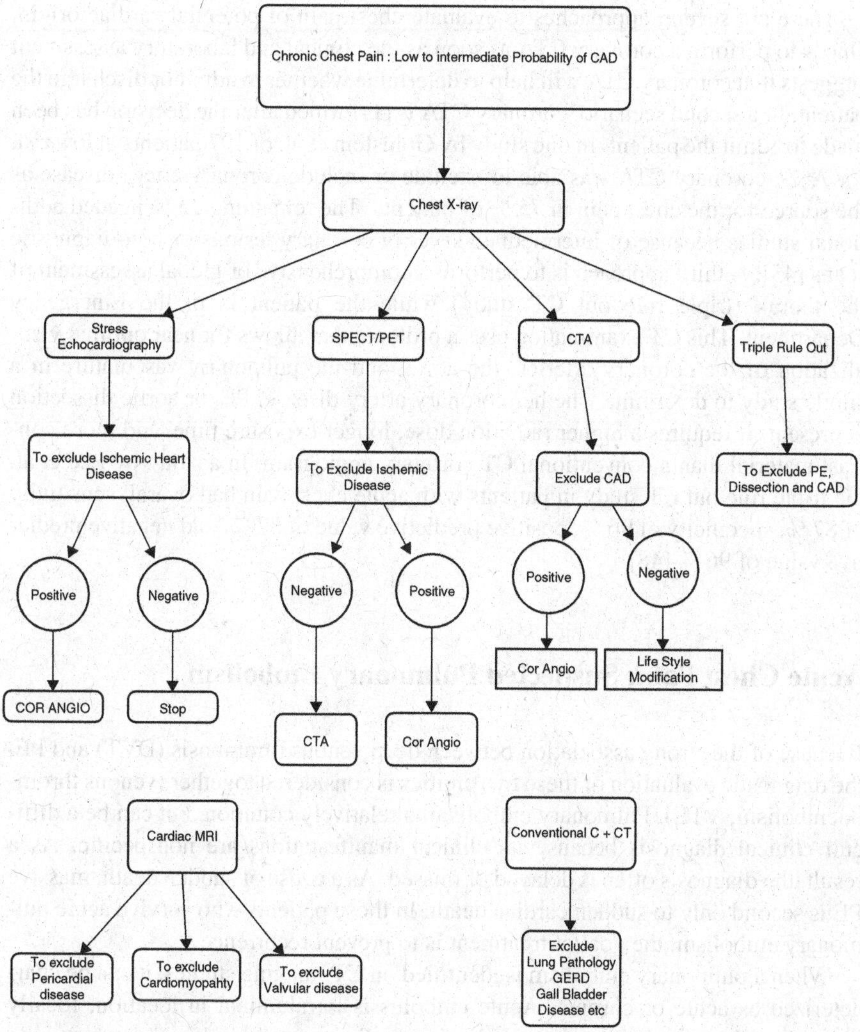

Fig. 3.7 Evaluation of chronic chest pain

The current generation of MDCT scanners units permits excellent resolution of cardiac structures. Although they have only one third of the resolution of catheter coronary arteriography, MDCT can visualize vessels of less than 2 mm in diameter. Studies show better than 80 % specificity for the determination of abnormal coronary artery morphology compared with intra-arterial coronary arteriography [45, 46].

CT without contrast enhancement can be used to quantify calcium load and hence the severity of atherosclerosis in the coronary arteries. This examination is used primarily for screening and shows good correlation with the incidence of subsequent acute cardiac events. An absence of coronary calcium has a high negative predictive value for the prediction of significant coronary artery disease [47].

There are several approaches to evaluate chest pain of potential cardiac origin. One is to perform a coronary CTA as soon as the clinical and laboratory assessment suggests that coronary CTA will help to determine whether to admit or discharge the patient. In a second scenario, coronary CTA is performed after the decision has been made to admit the patient. In one study by Goldstein et al. of 197 patients at low risk for ACS, coronary CTA was able to exclude or include coronary artery disease as the source for the chest pain in 75 % of patients. The remaining 25 % needed additional studies because of intermediate severity coronary lesions or non-diagnostic scans [45]. A third approach is to perform a comprehensive or global assessment of the thorax (triple rule out CT study) while the patient is in the Emergency Department. This CT examination uses a protocol that allows for near optimal visualization of the coronary arteries, the aorta, and the pulmonary vasculature in a single study to determine whether coronary artery disease, PE, or aortic dissection is present. It requires a higher radiation dose, longer exposure time, and more contrast material than a conventional CT coronary angiogram. In a study by Lee et al. the triple rule out CT study in patients with acute chest pain had overall sensitivity of 87 %, specificity of 96 %, positive predictive value of 87 %, and negative predictive value of 96 % [48].

Acute Chest Pain: Suspected Pulmonary Embolism

Because of the strong association between deep venous thrombosis (DVT) and PE, the diagnostic evaluation of these two entities is considered together (venous thromboembolism, VTE). Pulmonary embolism is relatively common, but can be a difficult clinical diagnosis because its clinical manifestations are nonspecific. As a result, the diagnosis often is delayed or missed. As a cause of sudden death, massive PE is second only to sudden cardiac death. In those patients who survive acute pulmonary embolism, the goal of treatment is to prevent recurrence.

When a pulmonary embolism is identified on CT imaging studies, it can be characterized as acute or chronic. Acute embolus is intraluminal in location, focally distending the vessel. Chronic embolus is usually eccentric in location, narrowing the arterial lumen and tapering the vessel diameter. Hemodynamic changes from pulmonary embolism are related to the embolic load, whether the emboli involve the central or peripheral vessels and the baseline cardiopulmonary status of the patient. Chronic pulmonary embolism is an important treatable cause of secondary pulmonary hypertension.

The imaging evaluation of PE aims to establish an acceptable level of diagnostic certainty of PE using the least invasive tests to warrant anticoagulant therapy while excluding other reasons for the patient's symptoms. Evidence-based literature supports the practice of determining the clinical probability (Wells Criteria) of PE before proceeding with diagnostic testing. The probability of a patient having PE is typically determined using a Bayesian approach in which the clinical (pre-test)

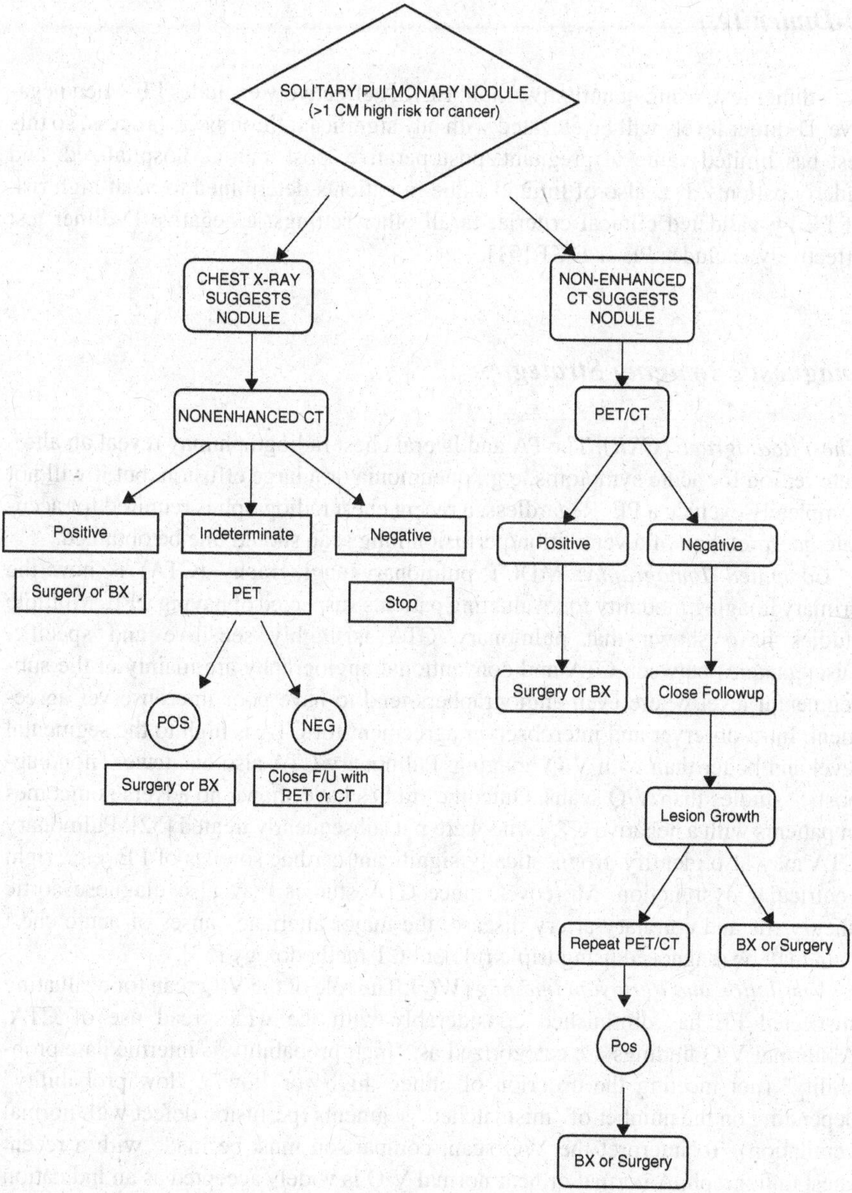

Fig. 3.8 Diagnostic imaging algorithm for pregnant patients suspected of PE

likelihood of PE, based on clinical criteria, is modified by the results of the appropriate radiological procedure(s) in order to estimate a post-test probability of PE. Figure 3.8 illustrates a practical algorithm for evaluating clinically suspected PE in nonpregnant patients who have no contraindication to intravenous contrast [49, 50].

D-Dimer Test

A D-dimer test, using quantitative rapid ELISA effectively excludes PE when negative. D-dimer levels will be elevated with any significant thrombotic process, so this test has limited value in pregnant, postoperative, post-trauma, hospitalized, and elderly patients. It is also of limited value in patients determined to be at high risk of PE by validated clinical criteria. In all other settings, a negative D-dimer test effectively excludes PE or DVT [51].

Diagnostic Imaging Strategies

Chest Radiograph (CXR): The PA and lateral chest radiograph may reveal an alternate reason for acute symptoms, e.g., pneumonia or a large effusion, but it will not completely exclude a PE. Regardless, a recent chest radiograph is required for accurate interpretation of a ventilation/perfusion lung scan should one be obtained.

Computed Tomography: MDCT pulmonary angiography (CTA) is now the primary imaging modality for evaluating patients suspected of having a PE. Multiple studies have shown that pulmonary CTA is highly sensitive and specific. Discrepancies between CTA and conventional angiography are mainly at the subsegmental level where even angiographers tend to have poor interobserver agreement. Intra-observer and interobserver agreement for CTA is high to the segmental level and better than with V/Q imaging. Pulmonary CTA also has fewer "nondiagnostic" studies than V/Q scans. Outcome studies have shown no adverse outcomes in patients with a negative CTA who were not subsequently treated [52]. Pulmonary CTA may also identify prognostically significant cardiac sources of PE, e.g., right ventricular dysfunction. Moreover, since CTA studies may also diagnose aortic aneurysms and coronary artery disease, the major alternate causes of acute chest pain may be diagnosed using triple rule out CT methodology [53].

Ventilation and Perfusion Imaging (V/Q): The role of the V/Q scan for evaluating suspected PE has diminished considerably with the widespread use of CTA. Abnormal V/Q findings are categorized as: "high probability," "intermediate probability" (not meeting the criterion of either "high" or "low"), "low probability" depending on the number of "mismatched" segments (perfusion defect with normal ventilation). To interpret the V/Q scan, comparison must be made with a recent chest radiograph. A normal or near normal V/Q is widely accepted as an indication that the patient has no PE and therefore no further workup for PE is necessary.

Lower Extremity Deep Venous Ultrasound: Because of the high association of DVT with PE, US evaluation (duplex Doppler with leg compression and spectral Doppler) of the venous drainage of the lower extremities is indicated in the evaluation of a patient for potential PE. The presence (or absence) of DVT does not indicate the presence (or absence) of PE, but significantly increases (or decreases) its

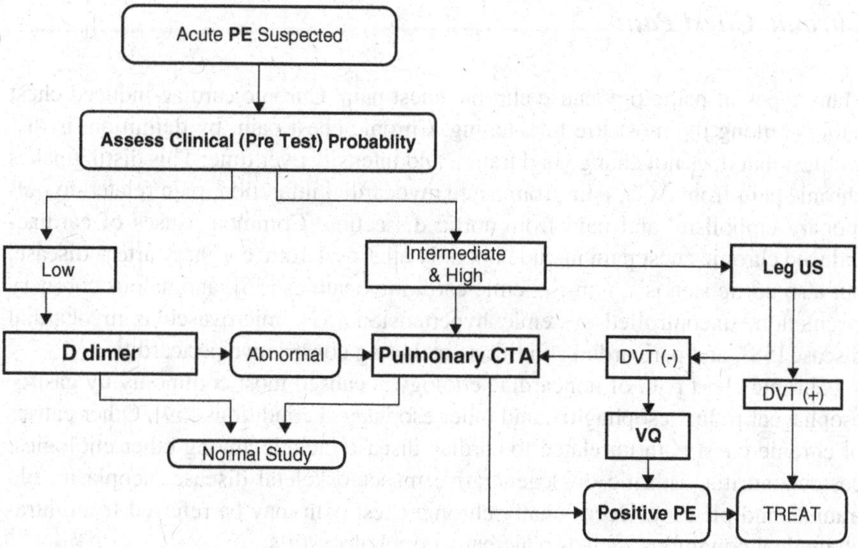

Fig. 3.9 MDCT-CTA centric diagnostic imaging algorithm for nonpregnant patients suspected of PE

likelihood. As not all pulmonary emboli originate from DVT in the lower extremities, a negative extremity US study does not exclude PE. A small proportion arises in the pelvic veins which cannot be visualized by US. Fewer yet arise in the deep veins of the upper extremity. Positive DVT studies may identify patients who are at high risk for recurrent PE and so are candidates for IVC filter placement. In most patients, however, the therapy for DVT, whether or not associated with PE, is identical to acute PE and consists of anticoagulation. Thus, no further diagnostic evaluation for PE is needed if DVT is identified.

Pregnancy and PE: Pregnancy is associated with a fivefold increase in the prevalence of DVT [54]. The risks of teratogenic effects of radiation militate against high-dose studies during pregnancy. Thus, the usual "first-line" examinations include a chest radiograph and lower extremity venous ultrasound. If these tests are non-diagnostic, a "second-line" examination, for example low-dose lung scintigraphy or low-dose pulmonary CTA, should be performed. Figure 3.9 illustrates a practical algorithm for evaluating pregnant patients who are suspected of having a PE.

The safety profile of gadolinium during pregnancy has not been established and so MR with IV contrast is not performed during pregnancy. In the future, non-contrast MR pulmonary arteriography may become an attractive alternative to CTA in pregnant patients. On the other hand, MR venography (MRV) can be performed without intravenous contrast and is both more accurate than US in the detection of lower extremity venous thrombosis and better than US in assessing the IVC and pelvic veins [55].

Chronic Chest Pain

Many types of pathology cause chronic chest pain. Chronic cardiac-induced chest pain is among the most life-threatening. Chronic chest pain, by definition, is discomfort that does not change in duration and intensity over time. This distinguishes chronic pain from ACS, pain from acute myocardial infarction, pain related to pulmonary embolism, and pain from aortic dissection. Common causes of cardiac-induced chronic chest pain include not only atherosclerotic coronary artery disease, but also aortic stenosis, non-ischemic cardiomyopathies [56], anomalous coronary circulation, uncontrolled systemic hypertension [57], microvascular myocardial disease [58], and pericardial conditions including constrictive pericarditis.

Chronic chest pain of noncardiac etiology is caused most commonly by gastroesophageal reflux, esophagitis, and other esophageal conditions [59]. Other causes of chronic chest pain unrelated to cardiac disease include among other etiologies: costochondritis, arthritic or degenerative musculoskeletal disease, neoplasm, old trauma, and pleurisy. Occasionally chronic chest pain may be referred from intra-abdominal conditions such as pancreatitis or cholecystitis.

The first step in evaluating a patient with chronic chest pain is to determine the clinical probability that the cause is coronary artery disease. This judgment requires assessment as to whether the chest pain is typical angina, atypical angina or noncardiac pain and comparing these symptoms with the patient's age, risk factors, and a variety of laboratory and imaging diagnostic criteria [60].

If the probability of coronary artery disease is intermediate or high, i.e., greater than 50 % in the clinician's estimation, the patient should undergo a cardiac evaluation (Fig. 3.7). This usually includes a chest X-ray and a resting EKG as base line studies followed by stress physiology assessment, either exercise echocardiography for myocardial contractility assessment, thallium radionuclide stress examination, or a stress single photon emission CT myocardial perfusion imaging evaluation (SPECT) [61]. MRI may also be helpful. A cardiac stress test is designed to provoke perfusion and/or contractility abnormalities. The stress may be exercise- or pharmacologically induced. Recently, PET has begun to replace SPECT because of its superior spatial resolution [62]. If a stress-related study is positive, there is a high probability of significant coronary artery disease, and the patient should be considered as a candidate for cardiac catheterization [63]. If aortic stenosis or if pericardial disease is thought to be the etiology of the chest pain, a resting echocardiogram should be performed. Patients, who after stress evaluation have equivocal results for CAD, should go onto a coronary CTA. This study has the advantage of ease of performance, high negative predictive value for the exclusion of coronary artery disease, and modest radiation dose when performed with the latest equipment and techniques [64]. Coronary CTA can also detect a variety of other cardiac-related conditions, including anomalous coronary circulation, pericardial disease, coronary bypass graft occlusion, and left ventricular contractility abnormalities. If it is done as part of a triple rule out study, pulmonary thromboembolism and aortic dissection can be excluded as alternative causes of chest pain. Of course, both of these conditions are usually causes of acute rather than chronic chest pain.

When echocardiography or radionuclide studies are non-diagnostic or equivocal, MRI either alone or with dobutamine or adenosine stress may be useful in the evaluation of chronic chest pain. Cardiac MRI without pharmacologic stress is useful to evaluate valvular and pericardial disease, cardiac neoplasm, and non-ischemic conditions such as hypertrophic obstructive cardiomyopathy and cardiac amyloidosis. Stress MRI may provide high sensitivity and specificity for the presence of ischemic myocardial disease by the induction of ventricular wall abnormalities [65].

Chronic Chest Pain of Probable Noncardiac Etiology

Those patients with chronic chest pain whose clinical evaluation and risk factors suggest a noncardiac etiology should have a standard two-view chest radiographic study. This can help to exclude a number of conditions including osseous pathology, lung cancer, and other chest masses. It may also show other diseases whose symptoms the patient may interpret as chronic chest pain, e.g., interstitial lung disease, emphysema, hiatus hernia, pleural disease, and sarcoidosis.

Gastroesophageal reflux disease (GERD) is the most common cause of noncardiac chronic chest pain and found in up to 60 % of such patients [66, 67]. In these patients, a barium study, pH monitoring, or endoscopy are studies of choice. Beyond a workup for gastroesophageal disease, the imaging algorithm should depend on the clinical history and the patient's signs and symptoms. For example, a chest CT should be obtained to exclude a lung mass in the patient with chest pain, cough, and weight loss. A bone scan and appropriate X-rays should be obtained in a patient with a known malignancy and rib pain on palpation. Chronic pulmonary emboli may be a cause of chest discomfort and in those patients where chronic pulmonary emboli is suspected a CT pulmonary angiogram, or if the patient has a contraindication to iodinated contrast, a V/Q study as an alternative should be pursued (Table 3.5).

Table 3.5 Evaluation of chronic non-anginal pain

1. The patient's risk factors for CAD should be determined
2. Is the chronic chest pain anginal in character?
3. If there is low to intermediate clinical probability for CAD and the chest pain is determined to be non-anginal, further testing should be based on the patient's signs and symptoms
4. GERD is the most common cause of noncardiac chest pain, a barium swallow examination, endoscopy, manometry, or esophageal pH studies may be most appropriate. Imaging may include assessment for non-coronary artery cardiac disease, e.g., CTA for ventricular function, echocardiography for valvular or pericardial disease, and/or MRI for infiltrative or hypertrophic cardiomyopathies
5. If the cause of the chronic chest pain remains an enigma, chest CT may be useful to exclude lung tumor, chronic pleural disease, and a host of other cardiothoracic conditions

Thoracic Aortic Aneurysm

About 25 % of aortic aneurysms occur in the thoracic aorta. Of these, approximately 60 % involve the aortic root and/or ascending aorta. The majority of ascending aortic aneurysms are associated with degenerative changes in the elastic layer of the aorta (cystic medial necrosis), and they are generally fusiform in shape. The combination of dilatation of the aortic root and the proximal ascending aorta with effacement of the sinotubular junction is termed annuloaortic ectasia. Annuloaortic ectasia may occur as an isolated condition or as part of a generalized disorder of connective tissue such as Marfan syndrome.

In contrast, the majority of descending aortic aneurysms are associated with atherosclerosis. They can be fusiform, saccular, or irregular in shape. A major consequence of thoracic aortic aneurysm (TAA) is aortic dissection or rupture (acute aortic syndrome, AAS). Patients with dissection typically complain of pain radiating to their back while those with rupture may have similar complaints if the rupture is contained. The goals of imaging in these patients include measurement of the maximum diameter, the craniocaudal extent of the aneurysm, aortic branch vessel involvement, extent of mural thrombus, identification of any impending signs of rupture, and evaluation of any periaortic pathology [68, 69].

Imaging the Thoracic Aortic Aneurysm

Chest Radiograph (CXR): CXR is insensitive for the detection of small TAA. The mediastinum may obscure an aneurysm completely, and so the chest X-ray may appear normal. Of course, CXR is not useful for identification of dissection or rupture.

Multidetector Computed Tomogram (MDCT): CTA is particularly useful in the evaluation of aortic aneurysms. It provides a comprehensive evaluation of the anatomy of the entire aorta and the renal, mesenteric, and iliac arteries. Non-contrast MDCT done prior to CTA can show acute hemorrhage into the wall of the aorta in a dissection. It is excellent at defining the shape and extent of the aneurysm, and its anatomic relationship to the visceral and renal vessels. Disadvantages include cost, use of ionizing radiation, and the risk of a hypersensitivity reaction to intravenous contrast media. High accuracy in sizing aneurysms makes CTA an excellent modality for serially monitoring changes in aneurysm size [70].

Echocardiography: TTE is a simple inexpensive noninvasive way of studying the left ventricular outflow tract, aortic root, and the proximal ascending aorta for annuloaortic ectasia. TTE can easily detect aortic insufficiency and aneurysms of the sinus of Valsalva. In stable patients, MDCT or MRI is preferred over TEE, which is mildly invasive, to image the thoracic aorta that cannot be visualized by TTE. TEE may be useful in patients who cannot receive intravenous iodinated contrast to show the aortic wall in greater detail than is possible with TTE [71].

Magnetic resonance imaging (MRI): MRI and MRA can accurately show the location, extent, and size of an aortic aneurysm as well as its relationship to branch vessels and surrounding organs. To avoid high exposure to radiation and multiple doses of intravenous contrast, MRI is preferred over MDCT/CTA when multiple follow-up studies are expected (particularly in younger patients) as well as in patients with compromised renal function.

Catheter Aortography and Selective Arteriography: Intra-arterial catheter aortography can delineate the aortic and branch vessel lumen, but does not help in defining the size of the aneurysm because this technique does visualize only the lumen of the vessel and not the outer diameter. On the other hand, selective arteriography can evaluate coronary anatomy, ventricular function by ventriculography, and aortic valvular insufficiency. Thus, catheter angiography and aortography can be useful in treatment planning. Today, because of its invasive nature, this study has become a backup examination to CTA or is used when therapeutic stenting is contemplated.

Surveillance: Serial Imaging

Patients with aortic aneurysms should have serial imaging to identify signs of impending or contained rupture. The imaging interval may vary from 6 months to a year. Of course, if there is a significant increase in aneurysm size from one study to the next, the interval between studies should be decreased. Note that MDCT and MRI measure the external diameter of the aneurysm. The resulting measurement is expected to be 0.2–0.4 cm larger than the TTE/TEE measured internal diameter. It is strongly recommended that the same modality be used consistently for follow-up imaging.

The rate of TAA enlargement varies, and the threshold size for elective intervention differs depending on the aneurysm's etiology, location, and associated symptoms:

- Ascending aorta: >4.5 cm for Marfan, >5.5 cm for atherosclerotic aneurysm.
- Aortic arch and descending aorta >5.5 cm.
- Thoracoabdominal aorta >6 cm.
- Growth rate >0.5 cm/year.
- Symptomatic with any size.

After operative repair of an aneurysm surveillance is performed at 1, 3, 6, and 12 months and then annually thereafter. Although the anatomical detail provided by CT may be better than that of MR in many instances, MRI and MRA are adequate for surveillance in stable patients [72].

Acute Aortic Syndrome

AAS describes a spectrum of life-threatening non-traumatic acute aortic pathology, including aortic dissection (AD), intramural hematoma (IMH), and penetrating atherosclerotic ulcer (PAU). Each of these conditions can lead to aneurysm formation and aortic rupture. The clinical manifestations of these conditions overlap. Sudden onset of severe sharp pain ("aortic pain") is the single most common presenting complaint. Pulse deficits and syncope are well-recognized signs often indicating branch hypoperfusion [73, 74].

Radiography: Chest radiography is performed routinely and can show widening of the mediastinum, widening and poor definition of the aortic contour, displaced aortic wall calcification, opacification of the aorticopulmonary window, and pleural effusion. However, 10–20 % of patients have a completely normal chest radiograph.

ECG: An ECG must be performed in all patients with suspected AAS. ECG helps to differentiate AAS from ACS. These two entities have different therapies with anticoagulation often indicated in ACS. In contrast, anticoagulation is contraindicated in AAS. Furthermore, both ACS and AAS may coexist.

MDCT/CTA: Catheter aortography, previously considered the test of choice for AAS, is rarely performed today. MDCT/CTA is currently the most frequently ordered test for the definitive diagnostic evaluation (Fig. 3.10). Non-contrast CT should be performed prior to CTA to look for intramural or false lumen acute hemorrhage. Typically, this is obscured by contrast administration. In addition, should ACS be suspected, CTA can be used to evaluate the coronary arteries. CT can assess the extent of aortic involvement and also depict involvement of visceral and iliac arteries. Unless the aorta has intimal calcification, differentiation between an aneurysm with mural thrombus and a dissection with a thrombosed false lumen can be difficult. Currently, CTA cannot assess for aortic insufficiency.

Imaging has the following goals:

- Confirmation of the diagnosis.
- Localization of the origin of an aortic tear.
- Extent and classification of aortic dissection and intramural hematoma.
- Great vessel and side-branch artery involvement.
- Identification of indicators for emergency surgery, e.g., pericardial, mediastinal, or pleural hemorrhage.

Echocardiography: Echocardiography is the second most commonly used tool in the initial diagnosis of AAS. TTE is paramount in assessing cardiac complications of dissection, including aortic insufficiency, pericardial tamponade, and regional and global left ventricular systolic and diastolic function. TTE is useful in diagnosing proximal aortic dissection, particularly when a type A dissection is suspected in a patient in shock since TTE may be performed portably at the bedside. TTE is limited, however, in visualizing the rest of the thoracic aorta.

Although TEE requires esophageal intubation, it is portable and can be performed at bedside. It can show intimal tears and differentiate between the true and false lumen of the aneurysm. TEE also can identify IMH and atherosclerotic penetrating ulcers. TEE requires the use of conscious sedation and should be avoided in patients with certain esophageal diseases [75, 76].

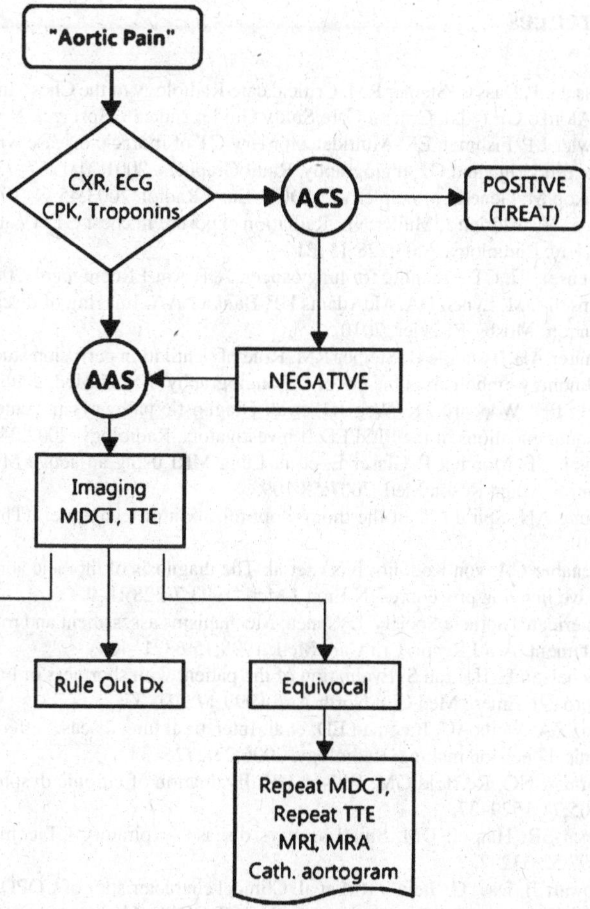

Fig. 3.10 Diagnostic imaging algorithm for evaluating patients presenting with pain suspected to be of aortic origin

MRI: MRI is a highly accurate diagnostic tool for detection of acute aortic dissection. Because of the limited availability of MRI, especially on an emergent basis, and the issues surrounding patient inconvenience and limited applicability (MRI cannot be performed on patients with claustrophobia, pacemakers, aneurysm clips, or other metal devices), MRI is used as a second line diagnostic study when the initial imaging study is inadequate. MRI helps to assess the age of the blood products in the wall in intramural hematoma. Even without contrast administration, flow in the false lumen can be analyzed using flow-sensitive sequences. MRI also can be used to quantitate aortic valve insufficiency and is also the modality of choice for repeated follow-up studies, particularly in younger patients.

References

1. Boiselle P, Dass C, Steiner RM. Critical care Radiology of the Chest. In Criner G, Barnette RE, D'Alonzo GE (eds). Critical Care Study Guide, 2nd edn. Springer, New York; 2010.
2. Lawler LP, Fishman EK. Multidetector row CT of thoracic disease with emphasis on 3D volume rendering and CT angiography. RadioGraphics. 2001;21:1257–73.
3. Prokop M. General principles of MDCT. Eur J Radiol. 2003;45:s4–10.
4. Mayo JR, Aldrich J, Muller NL. Radiation exposure in chest CT: a statement of the Fleischner Society. Radiology. 2003;228:15–21.
5. Swensen SJ. CT screening for lung cancer. AJR Am J Roentgenol. 2002;179:733.836.
6. Hansell DM, Lynch DA, McAdams HP, Bankier AA. Imaging of diseases of the chest 5th ed. London: Mosby-Elsevier; 2010.
7. Maurer AH, Tweddle B, Steiner RM. Role of ventilation perfusion studies for the diagnosis of pulmonary embolism in the era of CT angiography. J Nucl Med. 2006;47:21.
8. Stein PD, Woodard PK, Weg JG, et al. Diagnostic pathways in acute pulmonary embolism: recommendations of the PIOPED II investigators. Radiology. 2007;242:15–21.
9. Arnold JF, Morchel P, Glaser E, et al. Lung MRI using an active MR-compatible breathing control. Magn Reson Med. 2007;58:1092.
10. Leung AN. Spiral CT, of the thorax: optimization of technique. J Thorac Imaging. 1997;12: 2–10.
11. Nienaber CA, von Kodolitsch NV, et al. The diagnosis of thoracic aortic dissection by noninvasive imaging procedures. N Engl J Med. 1993;7(328):1–9.
12. American Thoracic Society. Dyspnea: Mechanisms assessment and management: a consensus statement. Am J Respir Crit Care Med. 1999;159:321–40.
13. Michelson E, Hollrah S. Evaluation of the patient with shortness of breath: an evidence based approach. Emerg Med Clin North Am. 1999;17:221–37.
14. Aziz ZA, Wells AU, Bateman ED, et al. Interstitial lung disease: effects of thin section CT on clinical decision making. Radiology. 2006;238:725–33.
15. Karnani NG, Reisfeld GM, Wilson GR. Evaluation of chronic dyspnea. Am Fam Physician. 2005;71:1529–37.
16. Desai SR, Hansell DM. Small airways disease: expiratory CT comes of age. Clin Radiol. 1997;52:332–7.
17. Stewart JI, Dass C, Steiner RM et al. Clinical characteristics of COPD patients: comparison of phenotype patterns of emphysema on MDCT COPD:2013 (in press).
18. Tocino I. Pneumothorax in the supine patient: radiographic anatomy. Radiographics. 1985;4: 557–85.
19. Lesur O et al. Computed tomography in the etiologic assessment of idiopathic spontaneous pneumothorax. Chest. 1990;98:341–7.
20. Omar H et al. Occult pneumothorax, revisited. J Trauma Manag Outcomes. 2010;4:12.
21. Lisenmeier U, Krotz M, Hauser H, et al. Whole body computed tomography in polytrauma. Eur Radiol. 2002;12:1728–40.
22. Wanek S, Mayberry JC. Blunt thoracic trauma. Crit Care Clin. 2004;20:71–81.
23. Shanmuganathan K, Mirvis SE. Imaging diagnosis of non-aortic thoracic injury. Radiol Clin North Am. 1999;37:533–61.
24. Trupka A, Wydhas C, Hallfedt KK, et al. Value of thoracic computed tomography in the first assessment of severely injured patients with blunt chest trauma: results of a prospective study. J Trauma. 1997;43:405.
25. Patel NH, Stephens, KE, Mirvis SE et al. Imaging of acute aortic injury due to blunt trauma: a review Radiology 1998:209:335-348).
26. Mirvis SE. Imaging in trauma and critical care. 2nd ed. Saunders Philadelphia 2003.
27. Lochum S, Ludig T, Walter F, et al. Imaging of diaphragmatic injury: a diagnostic challenge. Radiographics. 2002;22:S103–16.

28. Franquet T, Gimenez A, Akegret X, et al. Imaging findings of sternal abnormalities. Eur Radiol. 1997;7:492–7.
29. Paytel E, Menegaux F, Cluzel P, et al. Initial injury assessment of severe blunt trauma. Intensive Care Med. 2001;27:1756–61.
30. Holloway BJ, Rosewarne D, Jones RG, et al. Imaging of thoracic aortic disease. Br J Radiol. 2011;84:S338–54.
31. Mosquera VX, Marini M, Gulías D, et al. Minimal traumatic aortic injuries: meaning and natural history. Interact Cardiovasc Thorac Surg. 2012;14:773–8.
32. Mundy IM, Auwaerter PG, Oldach D, et al. Community-acquired pneumonia: impact of immune status. Am J Respir Crit Care Med. 1995;152:1309–15.
33. Brooks SW, Young JC, Cmolik B, et al. The use of TEE in the evaluation of chest trauma. J Trauma. 1992;32:761–5.
34. Hossack KE, Moreno CA, Vanway CW, et al. Frequency of cardiac contusion in nonpenetrating chest injury. Am J Cardiol. 1988;61:391.
35. Revel MP, Fournier LS, Hennebique AS, et al. Can CT replace bronchoscopy in the detection of the site and cause of bleeding in patients with large or massive hemoptysis? AJR Am J Roentgenol. 2002;179:1217–24.
36. Klein J, Braff S. Imaging evaluation of the solitary pulmonary nodule. Clin Chest Med. 2008;29:5–38.
37. MacMahon H, Austin JH, Gamsu G, et al. Guidelines for the management of small pulmonary nodules detected on CT scans. Radiology. 2005;237:395.
38. White CS, Kuo D. Chest pain in the emergency department: role of multidetector CT. Radiology. 2007;245:672–80.
39. Donat WE. Chest pain: cardiac and noncardiac causes. Clin Chest Med. 1987;8:241–52.
40. McCraig LF, Burt CS. National hospital ambulatory medical care survey: 2003 emergency department survey. Advanced data from vital and health statistics No 358. Hyattsville, MD: National Center for Health; 2005.
41. Stanford W, Levin DC, Bettman MA et al. Acute Chest Pain: no ECG evidence of Myocardial/ Infarction. American College of Radiology Appropriateness Criteria. Radiology 2000;215 Suppl 79–84h Statistics 2005.
42. Johnson TN, Nikolaou K, Wintersperger BJ, et al. ECG-gated 64 MDCT angiography in the differential diagnosis of acute chest pain. AJR Am J Roentgenol. 2007;188:76–82.
43. Urbania TH, Hope MD, Huffaker SD, Reddy GP. Role of computed tomography in the evaluation of acute chest pain. J Cardiovasc Comput Tomogr. 2009;3 Suppl 1:513–22.
44. Goldman L, Kirtane AJ. Triage of patients with acute chest pain and possible cardiac ischemia: The elusive search for diagnostic perfection. Ann Intern Med. 2003;139:987–95.
45. Hoffman U, Nagurney JT, Moselewski F, et al. Coronary multidetector computed tomography in the assessment of patients with acute chest pain. Circulation. 2006;114:2251–60.
46. Goldstein JA, Gallagher MJ, O'Neill WW, et al. A randomized controlled trial of multi-slice coronary computed tomography for evaluation of acute chest pain patients. J Am Coll Cardiol. 2007;49:863.871.
47. Greenland P, Bonow RO, Brundage BH, et al. ACCF/AHA 2007 clinical expert consensus document on coronary artery calcium scoring by computed tomography in global cardiovascular risk assessment and in evaluation of patients with chest pain. J Am Coll Cardiol. 2007; 49:378–402.
48. Lee HY, Yoo SM, White CS. Coronary CT angiography in emergency department patients with acute chest pain: Triple rule out protocol vs. dedicated coronary CT angiography. Int J Cardiovasc Imaging. 2009;25:319–26.
49. Agnelli G, Becattini C. Current concepts: acute pulmonary embolism. N Engl J Med. 2010;363:266–74.
50. Sadigh G, Kelly AM, Cronin P. Challenges, controversies, and hot topics in pulmonary embolism imaging. AJR Am J Roentgenol. 2011 Mar;196(3):497–515.
51. Stein PD, Hull RD, Patel RD et al. D-dimer for the exclusion of venous thrombosis and pulmonary embolism: a systematic review. Ann Intern Med:2004:140:569-602.

52. Reinartz P, Wildberger JE, Schaefer W, et al. Tomographic Imaging for the diagnosis of pulmonary embolism: a comparison between V/Q lung scintography with SPECT technique and multislice spiral CT. J Nucl Med. 2004;45:1501–8.
53. Bettmann MA, Baginski SG, White RD et al. Expert Panel on Cardiac Imaging. ACR Appropriateness Criteria® acute chest pain—suspected pulmonary embolism. [online publication]. Reston, VA: American College of Radiology (ACR); 2011. p. 7.
54. Papinger I, Grafenhofer H. Anticoagulation during pregnancy. Semin Thromb Hemost. 2003; 29:633–8.
55. Duran-Mendicuti A, Sodickson A. Imaging evaluation of the pregnant patient with suspected pulmonary embolism. Int J Obstet Anesth. 2011;20(1):51–9.
56. O'Gara PT, Bonow RO, Maron BJ, et al. Myocardial perfusion abnormalities in patients with hypertrophic cardiomyopathy: assessment with thallium-201 emission tomography. Circulation. 1987;76:1214–23.
57. Prisant LM, von Dohlon TW, Houghton JL, et al. A negative thallium stress test excludes significant obstructive epicardial coronary artery disease in hypertensive patients. Am J Hypertens. 1992;5:71–5.
58. Diamond GA, Forrester JS. Analysis of probability as an aid in the clinical diagnosis of coronary artery disease. N Engl J Med. 1979;300:1350–8.
59. Kachintorn U. How do we define non-cardiac chest pain? J Gastroenterol Hepatol 2005; 20 Suppl:S 2–5.
60. Gibbons RJ, Balady GJ, Bricker JT, et al. ACC/AHA 2002 Guideline update for exercise testing: summary article. Circulation. 2002;106:1883–92.
61. Metz LD, Beattie M, Hom R, et al. The prognostic value of normal exercise myocardial perfusion imaging and exercise echocardiography: a meta-analysis. J Am Coll Cardiol. 2007;49: 227–37.
62. Yoshinaga J, Chow BJ, Williams K, et al. What is the prognostic value of myocardial perfusion imaging using rubidium-82 positron emission tomography? J Am Coll Cardiol. 2006;48: 1029–39.
63. Earls JP, White RD, Woodard PK, et al. ACR appropriateness criteria: chronic chest pain: high probability of coronary artery disease. J Am Coll Radiol. 2011;8:679–86.
64. Gerber T, Kantor B, McCollough CH. Radiation dose and safety in cardiac computed tomography. Cardiol Clin. 2009;37:665–77.
65. Hundley WG, Morgan TM, Neagle CM, et al. Magnetic resonance imaging determination of cardiac prognosis. Circulation. 2002;106:2328–33.
66. Ruigomez A, Masso-Gonzales EL, Johansson S, et al. Chest pain without established ischaemic heart disease in primary care patients: associated comorbidities and mortality. Br J Gen Pract. 2009;59:E78–86.
67. Kones R. Recent advances in the management of chronic stable angina I: approach to the patient, diagnosis, pathophysiology, risk stratification, and gender disparities. Vasc Health Risk Manag. 2010;6:635–56.
68. HiratzkaLF, Bakris GL, Beckman JA, et al. ACCF/AHA/AATS/ACR/ASA/SCA/SCAI/ SIR/ STS/ SVM guidelines for the diagnosis and management of patients with thoracic aortic disease. J Am Coll Cardiol, 2010;55:27-129.
69. Ramnath VS, Oh JK, Sundt III TM, et al. Acute aortic syndromes and thoracic aortic aneurysm. Mayo Clin Proc. 2009;84(5):465–81.
70. Agarwal PP, Chughtai A, Matzinger F, et al. Multidetector CT of thoracic aortic aneurysms. RadioGraphics. 2009;29:537–52.
71. Konstadt SN, Reich DL, Quintana C, Levy M. The ascending aorta: how much does transephophageal echocardiography see? Anesth Analg. 1997;78:240–8.
72. Cozijnsen L, Braam RL, Waalewijn RA, et al. What is new in dilatation of the ascending aorta? Review of current literature and practical advice for the cardiologist. Circulation. 2011;123: 924–8.
73. Tsai TT, Nienaber CA, Eagle KA. Acute aortic syndromes. Circulation. 2005;112(24): 3802–13.

74. Vilacosta I, Aragoncillo P, Cañadas V, et al. Acute aortic syndrome: a new look at an old conundrum. Heart. 2009;95(14):1130–9.
75. Neinaber CA, Spielmann RP, Von Rodolitsch Y, et al. Diagnosis of thoracic aorta dissection: magnetic resonance imaging versus transesophageal echocardiography. Circulation. 1992;85: 444–7.
76. Douglas PS, Khandherra B, Steinback RF. Appropriatness criteria for transthoracic and transesophageal echocardiography. J Am Coll Cardiol. 2007;50:187–204.

Chapter 4
Breast Imaging

Robert Bronstein, Dillenia Reyes, and Theresa Kaufman

Breast imaging is a clinical subspecialty within the larger field of radiology. One in eight American women will develop invasive breast cancer during their lifetime. According to the American Cancer Society's estimates, about 232,340 new cases of invasive breast cancer will be diagnosed in women in 2013, with approximately 40,000 deaths. There are projected to be additional 64,640 new cases of in situ (non-invasive) breast cancer [1]. Breast cancer is the second leading cause of cancer death in women behind only lung cancer. In recent years, increased publicity has made women acutely aware of the risk of developing this disease.

History of Breast Imaging

Efforts to use imaging to evaluate breast disease with radiography began shortly after Wilhelm Roentgen discovered X-rays. Despite all the efforts over the years, clinically effective use of mammography was not truly available until the 1960s. Besides radiography, many other modalities aimed at diagnosing breast cancer have been tried. Thermography was used in the 1950s purporting to measure heat emanating from breast tumors due to their neovascularity. This modality did not prove clinically effective, and although recent efforts have been made to reintroduce thermography, its effectiveness has not improved. Although some women still choose thermography because their breasts do not have to be compressed while performing a thermogram, it should not be used as a substitute for mammography [2]. Xeroradiography was introduced in the 1970s. In this technique, a plate coated with selenium rests on a thin layer of aluminum oxide. The X-ray beam passes through

R. Bronstein, M.D. • D. Reyes, M.D. • T. Kaufman, D.O. (✉)
Department of Radiology, Temple University Medical School,
Philadelphia, PA 19140, USA
e-mail: theresa.kaufman@gmail.com

W.R. Reinus (ed.), *Clinician's Guide to Diagnostic Imaging*,
DOI 10.1007/978-1-4614-8769-2_4, © Springer Science+Business Media New York 2014

the breast and strikes the selenium plate, causing a charge distribution on the plate. Then, as with a paper copier, the image formed on the charged plate is transferred to paper for display. While xeroradiography produced usable images, it required too much radiation, and image storage and reproducibility were significant problems.

By 1960s, mammography was considered clinically safe although the radiation dose to the breast and shielding were not as good as they are today. The radiation dose currently delivered from a two view analogue mammogram has been reduced to approximately 2.37 mGY [3], about the equivalent amount of ambient radiation one receives from the atmosphere in 3 months. At the time the reproducibility, safety, and relative ease of performance also helped to make mammography a more viable option.

While mammograms became more available in the 1960s, it took time for its utility to be understood and utilized by the public. It was not until the mid-1980s that screening programs started to be promoted and until the 1990s that breast cancer awareness exploded with a marked increase in fundraising and cancer research. From the early 1960s when only 10–15 % of women took advantage of mammography, the number of women having yearly screening increased to a high of approximately 75 % in the early 2000s. As a result of strict adherence to a program of yearly mammographic screening after age 40, breast cancer deaths in women between 40 and 50 years of age who are screened have decreased by as much as 26–29 % [4].

The original technique of screen film mammography (analogue) while extremely useful does have limitations. Penetrating through breast parenchyma, particularly in dense breasts, is problematic. Dense parenchyma makes it more difficult to see masses and discern faint calcifications. Compressing the breasts during mammography helps improve penetration and makes lesions more conspicuous. Still, analogue mammography was not ideal.

The need for better techniques led to development of full field digital mammography (FFDM) which is now state of the art. Digital mammography has slightly worse spatial resolution than analogue mammography, but has much improved contrast resolution, allowing for better visualization of calcifications. With a digital display, post-processed magnification is easy and allows a much closer look at all areas of the breast. In addition, digital images permit computer-aided detection (CAD) techniques where a computer marks areas in the breast that it perceives as a mass or calcifications for closer examination after initial interpretation. The radiation dose with digital mammography has decreased to an average of approximately 1.86 mGy per study [3]. Digitized images are transported easily on disc, an aid in our highly mobile society to radiologists who need to compare all old studies to the current one to make an accurate assessment of the current study.

The FDA approved tomosynthesis, the next innovation in breast imaging, for clinical use in 2011. This is essentially a digital tomogram of the breast allowing review of the mammogram in 1 mm "slices." Studies are being conducted currently to assess value of one-view tomosynthesis vs. two-view FFDM vs. one-view tomosynthesis in combination with FFDM. One recent study showed that one-view tomosynthesis had better sensitivity and negative predictive value than FFDM in patients with fatty or very dense breasts [5].

In the process of attempting continually to improve and refine abilities to diagnose breast cancer earlier, an increased ability to diagnose benign conditions confidently was a significant by-product. Today, breast imaging is a vital component of overall management of breast health and disease, helping to diagnose benign as well as malignant conditions.

Screening Recommendations

In 2009, the United States Preventive Services Task Force recommended that women begin having screening mammograms at age 50, with follow-up mammograms every 2 years thereafter. It also stated that breast self-examination should not be performed [5]. Although an authoritative body, the conclusions of this study were spurious, the result of a flawed meta-analysis of 20 years of retrospective data. As a result, the medical community has rejected the recommendations of this study.

Current breast screening guidelines and recommendations from the American College of Radiology and American Cancer Society are for women at average risk for developing breast cancer to have a baseline mammogram at age 40 with annual follow-up mammograms [1, 6]. Furthermore, these guidelines recommend that breast self-examination begin at age 20. No age has been specified at which to stop obtaining yearly mammograms. It had been suggested that yearly mammographic screening stop at age 85, but today longer life expectancy has made that recommendation obsolete.

There are specific indications to begin breast screening in women before age 40 [7]:

- Carriers of BRCA gene.
- Untested first-degree relatives (mother, sister, daughter) of known BRCA carrier.
- First-degree relative of a woman diagnosed before menopause with breast cancer. Screening should begin 10 years before the age at which the relative was diagnosed or between the ages of 25 and 30, whichever is later.
- Women who have received mantle radiation for Hodgkin's disease.
- Women with any previous biopsy showing atypical hyperplasia of any type (ductal, lobular, lobular carcinoma in situ).

Additional considerations that may prompt earlier commencement of breast screening:

- Family history of breast and epithelial ovarian cancer.
- Breast cancer in a male family member.
- At least two family members on the same side diagnosed with breast cancer.

The Radiologists' Role

Many women sent for mammograms are very anxious. A commonly held misconception is that having a mammogram is painful, and many women need encouragement to complete the procedure. The need for a breast biopsy magnifies a woman's anxiety.

Performing interventional procedures is a significant part of the specialty. These include stereotactic biopsy using mammograms as a guide, ultrasound-guided breast biopsies, MRI-guided biopsies, fine needle aspirations (FNAs), cyst and abscess drainage, needle localization of breast lesions as guide to the breast surgeon and occasional galactograms. This means that the radiologist works in close association with the patient's surgeon and is an active member of the clinical team. The radiologist should meet with the breast surgeon and the pathologist on a regular basis for "concordance conference." The breast images, pathologic slides, and clinical results of all patients who have had biopsies are reviewed. If pathological results are not concordant with expected results based on imaging and clinical picture, rebiopsy (preferably by a different modality) is recommended.

Breast Imaging Tools

Mammography is the gold standard of breast cancer diagnosis. Many other modalities play ancillary roles in the diagnosis of breast disease. These include ultrasound and magnetic resonance imaging (MRI), neither of which uses ionizing radiation, molecular breast imaging (MBI, BSGI, scintimammography), positron emission mammography (PEM), and PET scanning. With some exceptions, these modalities are rarely used as primary screening tools.

Mammography

Mammography is the primary test used for breast screening and diagnosis. Because of differences in the appearance of breast tissue from woman to woman and even side to side in each woman, there is no "normal" mammogram. Every woman's baseline mammogram is *her normal*, and all subsequent mammograms must be compared to her baseline and subsequent mammograms. Any significant changes from baseline or previous mammogram must be evaluated further.

Mammograms, whether analogue or digital (as with all radiographs), can only display five radiographic densities. From least dense to most dense these are air, fat, soft tissue including fluid, bone/calcium, and metal. Normal breast parenchyma is soft tissue density with abundant interlobular fat. Unfortunately, breast tumors, benign breast lesions, e.g., fibroadenomas, breast cysts, hematomas, and mesenchymal lesions (hamartoma, angiomyolipoma, phyloides tumors), and abscesses are all basically soft tissue density and so similar in density to normal breast tissue. Subtle differences in the density as well as perceived morphology and significant asymmetries with remaining breast tissue allow masses to be visualized, some seen better than others. Masses usually require at least one additional modality for further characterization, most frequently ultrasound. This helps provide a more detailed analysis and ultimately either a diagnosis or a decision to biopsy.

- Mammograms are done either for screening or for a diagnostic evaluation. Screening mammograms consist of two views of each breast. Diagnostic mammograms are reserved for women with known breast-related complaints or with suspected lesions not fully evaluated on the initial mammogram. Both examinations begin with an interview by the technologist about the patient's personal breast history.
- Screening mammograms are read later by the radiologist after which an official report is generated with recommendations for next necessary study.
- Diagnostic mammograms are reviewed by the radiologist while the patient is present in the mammography suite and as many additional views as required are obtained to evaluate the patient's problem. If the patient has a palpable lesion, typically an ultrasound is performed on the same day.
- Radiologists miss at least 10 % of breast cancers on mammography, particularly in women with dense breasts [8]. This means that all women with palpable lesions should have an ultrasound regardless of mammography findings.

Men who complain of swelling in one or both breasts also may require mammography, although it is usually better to begin evaluation with ultrasound. Most often male breast swelling is caused by gynecomastia, but breast cancer does occur in males and has the same mammographic findings as seen in female breast cancer.

Mammography reporting is standardized according to the Breast Imaging and Data Reporting System (BIRADS) system. This system was developed in an attempt to have uniform reporting throughout the country. It makes recommendations for additional evaluation and so also serves the purpose of guiding the ordering clinician in the patient's workup. There are seven BIRADS categories [9]:

0. Further study needed (additional views, ultrasound, MRI).
1. Normal study. Recommend yearly follow-up mammogram.
2. Benign finding. Recommend yearly follow-up mammogram.
3. Probably benign finding. Recommend short-term (6 months) follow-up.
4. Malignancy suspected. Biopsy recommended.
   (May be subcategorized from A to C, according to increasing likelihood of malignancy.)
5. Malignancy strongly suspected (95 % certainty). Biopsy recommended.
   (Also may have A, B, and C subcategories.)
6. Malignancy diagnosed but not fully treated. Often used for follow-up to neoadjuvant chemotherapy.

Tomosynthesis

Mammography is a projectional technique, depicting the entire three-dimensional (3D) breast volume in two dimensions. Tomosynthesis acquires 3D thin-section data. Images can be reconstructed in the conventional orientations of mammography. Adding tomosynthesis to mammography permits improved evaluation of the borders of a mass, architectural distortion within the breast parenchyma, and the extent of microcalcifications within the tissue. It also permits 3D localization for surgical planning [10].

Ultrasound

Because ultrasound (US) gives no ionizing radiation, it can be used more liberally than mammography and is preferred in younger patients. Ultrasound also can penetrate dense breast tissue. Not only is ultrasound able to penetrate the dense breast tissue better than mammography, but it images thin "slices" of tissues at different depths in the breast. This means that it shows detail in a limited volume of the breast. As such it is a problem solving technique that allows differentiation of solid and cystic lesions. Today, with improved gray scale imaging and better displays, some differential characteristics of solid masses also can be discerned.

Recently, an automated breast ultrasound screening machine (ABUS) has been approved by the FDA. Currently, ABUS is not reimbursed by insurance companies. The American College of Radiology Imaging Network (ACRIN) published a study in April, 2012 showing that adding annual screening ultrasound to mammography in women with high breast cancer risk and dense breast tissue gave an incremental cancer detection rate of 3.7 per 1,000 women screened [11]. The breast cancers detected only by ultrasound have been small invasive cancers with a high proportion of node negative cases. The addition of screening ultrasound also resulted in increased false-positive rates that resulted in further investigation and biopsy. Ultrasound does not replace mammography for routine screening since currently mammography is the only imaging modality that has been proven to reduce mortality from breast cancer. ABUS might be considered effective enough in the future to be used as a screening tool.

To avoid exposure to ionizing radiation in younger women, ultrasound should be used as the primary tool of breast diagnosis only in women under 30 years-of-age who present with a palpable mass. Mammography may be required after the ultrasound if further characterization of the lesion is needed. Ultrasound is safe to use in pregnant women who not infrequently complain of new masses in their breasts, which are radically changed by the elevated hormone levels of pregnancy.

Ultrasound often is used as a guide to perform percutaneous biopsies of mammographically or ultrasonically detected abnormalities. These can be performed safely on an outpatient basis.

Elastography

Elastography is a new tool in the ultrasound armamentarium. This technique compares signals of a tissue before and after displacement using compression strain imaging, vibration sonoelastography, acoustic radiation force generated by the ultrasound pulse, and real-time shear waves to characterize the hardness or stiffness of a lesion. Malignancies tend to be less deformable than benign lesions, and so elastography can provide additional clues as to the character of a mass [12].

Magnetic Resonance Imaging

A recent addition to the armamentarium of the breast imager is magnetic resonance imaging (MRI). This modality uses no ionizing radiation, but rather uses high strength magnetic fields to polarize protons. The imaging can be acquired and displayed in multiple planes and tissue thicknesses. This allows for thin cross-sectional examination of breast tissue with excellent soft tissue contrast. Sagittal images are performed both before and after gadolinium injection with five 1.5–2 min sequentially obtained acquisitions after the initial postinjection imaging. The pre-contrast images are then subtracted from the post-contrast images to highlight areas of true enhancement. Sequential images from identical locations within the breast are studied for their rapidity of enhancement and subsequent dissipation of contrast to generate enhancement curves. The pattern of enhancement can provide clues as to the nature of a lesion [13]. As with mammography, CAD is available with MRI.

MRI is highly sensitive for mass detection, but overlap of the appearance and enhancement behavior is high and so MRI is not very specific. Early experience with MRI and MRI biopsies in a selected patient population by breast imagers at Sloane-Kettering led to the conclusion that enhancing lesions 5 mm or less should be followed rather than biopsied [14].

The high sensitivity and low specificity of MRI mean that, in general, it should not be used as a screening tool. Currently accepted indications for screening with MRI are:

- A young woman with dense breasts and a 20–25 % increased risk of breast cancer.
- Strong family history—two first-degree relatives or a male family member with breast cancer.
- BRCA carrier.
- Relative of a BRCA carrier.
- A positive axillary lymph node without a known primary (and normal mammogram).

The American Cancer Society (ACS) and the Society of Breast Imagers (SBI) guidelines state that screening MRI is inappropriate for women with less than a 15 % increased risk of developing breast cancer. In high-risk patients MRI can be alternated with mammography every 6 months or be performed yearly at the discretion of the radiologist and breast surgeon.

Otherwise, MRI is also employed to evaluate:

- The extent of disease preoperatively in a patient with known breast cancer.
- Tumor response to chemotherapy.
- For recurrence of tumor in an area of scarring.
- Breast implant leak or rupture.

Breast MRI should be performed between the third and fourteenth day of the woman's menstrual cycle to minimize background breast enhancement [12]. When abnormal areas of contrast enhancement are seen, breast ultrasound can be performed to see if the same lesion can be seen on US and therefore be biopsied with ultrasound guidance. Many MRI areas of enhancement are not mass-like and therefore cannot be seen on ultrasound. In these instances, MRI-guided biopsy is recommended.

It is not uncommon for the previously seen suspicious area of enhancement on MRI to have resolved when the patient returns for biopsy. This is a favorable finding since many physiologic changes can cause areas of MRI breast tissue enhancement. Enhancement from malignancies does not resolve, however. If suspicion persists despite disappearance of the enhancing region, a repeat MRI can be obtained in 6 months.

Molecular Breast Imaging (MBI, BSGI, Scintimammography)

Molecular breast imaging (MBI) was developed in the mid-1990s. Unlike other modalities that examine the breast anatomically, this modality measures cellular activity.

Breast-specific gamma imaging (BSGI) uses Tc^{99m} Sestamibi which accumulates in the mitochondria of the cells in direct correlation to the cellular energy conversion rate. Cancer cells produce more ATP from glucose than neighboring cells and so produce a hot spot on the BSGI image. When originally introduced, BSGI used a dose of 25 mCi of Tc^{99m} Sestamibi injected intravenously. This dose delivered too much radiation to the body and breast. Since then, improvements have been made including development of a dual headed scanner. This allowed the Sestamibi dose to be reduced to an acceptable 10 mCi and has the additional advantage or reducing examination time by half.

Another isotope currently available for nuclear breast scanning is flurodeoxyglucose (FDG) which is also used in traditional PET scans. FDG is less available than Sestamibi, requires the patient to fast overnight, and also must have a 1 h delay between injection and scanning. Care must also be used in diabetic patients. As a result Sestamibi is often the preferred radionuclide. Similar to MRI scanning, BSGI is ideally performed between the 2nd and 12th day of the menstrual cycle. Because the projections are the same as those performed in a routine mammogram, the two studies can and should be directly correlated, view by view.

The majority of breast cancers 5 mm or greater will accumulate isotope [15]. Tumors as small as 3 mm have been diagnosed using this technique. MBI is particularly good at detecting infiltrating lobular cancers. Multifocal and multicentric cancers may be detected as well.

As with MRI, BSGI is extremely sensitive, but has greater specificity than MRI. A recent study showed that BSGI can detect cancers missed by both mammography and ultrasound. In this study BSGI had the overall highest sensitivity (91 %) for breast cancer detection, much higher than mammography and ultrasound, 74 % and 84 %, respectively [16].

Entities beside breast cancer that show increased isotope uptake on BSGI include atypical ductal hyperplasia (ADH), papillomas, breast abscesses, and sclerosing adenosis. The negative predictive value of BSGI is 95–99 %, making it a valuable tool in breast cancer detection.

The indications for BSGI are similar to those for MRI and include evaluating the extent of disease in a patient with known breast cancer, monitoring response to chemotherapy, bloody nipple discharge, palpable abnormality with negative mammogram and ultrasound, positive axillary lymph node with no known primary tumor, patients with implants, patients with strong family history, and patients for whom MRI is contraindicated.

MBI has some limitations. Surgery may cause abnormal activity for up to a year. Lesions close to the chest wall or deep in the axilla may not be detected. One cannot adequately assess lesions adjacent to the chest wall or involving the chest wall. At least one company has developed a device capable of MBI directed biopsy.

Interventional Procedures

A number of diagnostic and therapeutic procedures, developed specifically for breast disease and all of which can be performed on an outpatient basis, have been developed. For biopsies, patient should be off all blood thinners and NSAIDs for 5–7 days.

Stereotactic Core Biopsy

This procedure uses a stereotactic pair of radiographs from which the location of the lesion within the breast can be calculated to within 0.1 mm in a single plane. This procedure is used primarily to biopsy suspicious calcifications and occasionally masses that are unreachable or not well-defined using US [17, 18].

The patient often lays prone on the biopsy table for stereotactic biopsy which may not be possible in patients with significant respiratory problems, scoliosis or arthritis, occasionally patients with pacemakers, or patients who have had recent surgery. For these people there are institutions that have erect stereotactic biopsy machines.

Ultrasound-Guided Breast Biopsy

Ultrasound can guide sterile biopsy of any lesion that cannot be called definitively benign, abnormal appearing lymph nodes and cysts that have mural nodules, thick walls, or internal solid components.

MRI-Guided Biopsy

This technique is used less commonly than US-guided biopsy because of the awkwardness of using an MR scanner, the time required to do the biopsy, the cost, and the inability to use in patients with internal ferromagnetic materials. It is used for lesions deemed suspicious on diagnostic MRI that cannot be seen on ultrasound.

Patients scheduled for any of the stereotactic, ultrasound, or MRI biopsy must have bleeding profiles as close to normal as possible. Warfarin and Plavix must be stopped for at least 5 days prior to biopsy. It is preferred that Aspirin and NSAIDs not be used for at least 1 week prior to biopsy.

Cyst and Abscess Aspiration

Simple cysts, i.e., smooth, thin wall; no mural thickening or nodules, are left alone unless the patient requests that they be aspirated. In 40 % of aspirated cysts the fluid will reaccumulate. Abscesses and cysts are drained under US guidance.

Fine Needle Aspiration

FNA is used primarily to biopsy abnormal appearing lymph nodes in a "tight" axilla (one with little fat where stereotactic core biopsy is not chosen because of close proximity of the axillary neurovascular bundle). The advantage of FNA is that it is quick and easy to perform. The drawback is that while differentiation between benignancy and malignancy often can be made, the amount of the tissue obtained using this technique is not enough to evaluate the hormonal status of malignant cells. Hence, another biopsy with a larger bore vacuum needle may be necessary [19].

Needle Localization for Breast Biopsy or Definitive Treatment of a Known Malignancy

Some suspicious microcalcifications cannot be assessed by stereotactic biopsy for technical reasons. In some cases a prior stereotactic biopsy failed, and a repeat biopsy is needed. Other patients who have had a positive biopsy return for definitive surgery. In these cases the target tissue will be difficult for a surgeon to find in operating room. A percutaneous localization is therefore performed. The radiologist, using imaging as guide, can put a needle with a hooked wire into the breast leaving its tip in the target area as a marker for the surgeon. The surgical specimen is sent for radiography to confirm that the target has been removed.

Galactography

Galactography is done to evaluate the intramammary ducts. Most often, this is done for patients with complaints of nipple discharge. Galactography requires cannulation of the duct orifice whence the discharge arises. Contrast is injected into the duct and radiographs of the opacified ducts are obtained and evaluated for intraductal lesions.

Clinical Scenarios

1. Palpable lump:
   (a) Patients under 35 years-of-age: Order ultrasound. You may also order mammogram if indicated allowing the radiologist the ability to order mammogram immediately if deemed necessary.
   (b) Patients over 35 years-of-age: Mammogram and ultrasound. Any woman complaining of a mass should have both a mammogram and ultrasound.
2. Inflamed, swollen breast with or without a palpable mass:
   (a) Start the patient on a 2-week course antibiotics when seen and obtain mammogram and ultrasound after the antibiotics course has been completed.
   (b) Both mastitis and inflammatory breast carcinoma will improve on antibiotics, but only mastitis will completely clear.
   (c) A punch biopsy of the skin is a quick and efficient way to biopsy since dermal lymphatics are involved in inflammatory carcinoma.
3. Breast pain:
   (a) Breast pain is a common complaint, but one that is unlikely to be related to cancer (other than inflammatory carcinoma).
   (b) Most women complain of breast pain at some time during her cycle—usually before menses.
   (c) If needed, obtain ultrasound in young women, ultrasound and/or mammogram in older women.

4. Mammogram shows indeterminate microcalcifications, asymmetric density(ies) or partially imaged lesion:
   (a) Obtain further views of that breast as recommended by the radiologist to better evaluate morphology. Any of these findings can arise from a malignancy.
   (b) If magnification views show calcifications to be suspicious, obtain stereotactic biopsy.
5. Palpable mass in a pregnant woman:
   (a) Obtain breast ultrasound.
   (b) Request mammogram per radiologist as necessary for further diagnosis. (All attempts are made to avoid mammography in pregnant patients.)
6. Male with palpable breast mass or swelling:
   (a) Obtain breast ultrasound and if necessary mammogram.
7. Patients who have had a breast biopsy, local excision, or partial mastectomy require a 6-month follow-up unilateral mammogram.
8. Patient complains of nipple inverting or a new skin dimple:
   (a) Obtain mammogram to study area beneath finding.
9. Patient with bloody or clear nipple discharge:
   (a) Obtain breast ultrasound in periareolar area, with possible mammogram at discretion of radiologist.
   (b) MRI might become necessary.
   (c) If these examinations fail to show the etiology of the discharge, a galactogam may be needed.
10. Breast reduction surgery planned:
    (a) Obtain mammogram as appropriate to the patient's age for surgical planning and to exclude cryptogenic disease.
11. Biopsy proven lobular carcinoma in situ (LCIS) (30 % lifetime increased breast cancer risk):
    (a) Patient needs wide excision of area.
    (b) More rigorous screening required either mammogram every 6 months, or mammogram alternating with MRI or BSGI every 6 months.
12. Ultrasound suggests fibroadenomas, *not* biopsied:
    (a) In younger woman (<30–35) biopsy or obtain 6-month follow-up ultrasounds for 2 years to assess lesion stability.
    (b) If first seen in woman over 35 or if growing in woman over 35, biopsy
13. Patient with 20 % increased risk of breast cancer
    (a) Start early breast screening with mammography (10 years before age at which first-degree relative was diagnosed.)

References

1. American Cancer Society. Breast cancer detailed guide. 2012. http://www.cancer.org/acs/groups/cid/documents/webcontent/003090-pdf.pdf. Accessed January 27, 2013.
2. U.S. Food and Drug Administration. FDA Safety Communication: Breast cancer screening-thermography is not an alternative to mammography. 2011. http://www.fda.gov/MedicalDevices/Safety/AlertsandNotices/ucm257259.htm. Accessed January 29, 2013.
3. Hendrick RE, Pisano ED, Averbukh A, Moran C, Burns E, et al. Comparison of acquisition parameters and breast dose in digital mammography and screen-film mammography in the American College of Radiology imaging network digital mammographic imaging screening trial. AJR Am J Roentgenol. 2010;194(2):362–9.
4. Tabar L, Vitac B, Chen TH, Cohen A, Tot T, et al. Swedish two county trial: impact of mammography screening on breast cancer mortality during 3 decades. Radiology. 2011;260(3):658–63.
5. Waldherr C, Cerny P, Altermatt HJ, Berclaz G, Ciriolo M, Buser K, Sonnenschein MJ. Value of one view tomosynthesis versus two-view mammography in diagnostic workup of women with clinical signs and symptoms and in women recalled from screening. AJR Am J Roentgenol. 2013;200(1):226–31.
6. U.S. Preventive Services Task Force. Screening for breast cancer recommendation statement. 2009. http://www.uspreventiveservicestaskforce.org/uspstf09/breastcancer/brcanrs.htm. Accessed January 29, 2013.
7. Mainiero MB, Lourenco A, Mahoney MC, Newell MS, Bailey L, et al. ACR appropriateness criteria breast cancer screening. JACR. 2013;10:11–4.
8. Humphrey LL, Helfand M, Chan BK, Woolf SH. Breast cancer screening: a summary of evidence for the U.S. preventive services task force. Ann Intern Med. 2002;137:347–60.
9. American College of Radiology. Breast imaging reporting and data system (BI-RADS). 4th ed. Reston, VA: American College of Radiology; 2003.
10. Park JM, Franken EA, Garg M, Fajardo LL, Niklason LT. Breast tomosynthesis: present considerations and future applications. Radiographics. 2007;27:S231–40.
11. Berg WA, Zhang Z, Lehrer D, Jong RA, Pisano ED, et al. Detection of breast cancer with addition of annual screening ultrasound or a single screening MRI to mammography in women with elevated breast cancer risk. JAMA. 2012;307(13):1394–404.
12. Ginat DT, Destounis S, Barr RG, Castaneda B, Strang JG, Rubens DJ. US elastography of breast and prostate lesions. Radiographics. 2009;29:2007–16.
13. Macura KJ, Ouwerkerk R, Jacobs MA, Bluemke DA. Patterns of enhancement on breast MR images: interpretation and imaging pitfalls. Radiographics. 2006;26:1719–34.
14. Liberman L, Mason G, Morris EA, Dershaw DD. Does size matter? Positive predictive value of MRI-detected breast lesions as a function of lesion size. AJR. 2006;186:426–30.
15. Lumachi F, Ferretti G, Povolato M, Marzola MC, Zucchetta P, Geatti O, Brandes AA, Bui F. Accuracy of technetium-99m Sestamibi scintimammography and x-ray mammography in premenopausal women with suspected breast cancer. Eur J Nucl Med. 2001;28:1776–80.
16. Weigert JM, Bertrand ML, Lanzkowsky L, Stern LH, Kieper DA. Results of a multicenter patient registry to determine the clinical impact of breast-specific gamma imaging, a molecular breast imaging technique. AJR Am J Roentgenol. 2012;198(1):W69–75.
17. Desrshaw DD, Liberman L. Stereotactic breast biopsy: indications and results. Oncology. 1998;12(6):907–16.
18. Parker SH, Lovin JD, Jobe WE, Luethke JM, Hopper KD, Yakes WF, Burke BJ. Stereotactic breast biopsy with a biopsy gun. Radiology. 1990;76:741–7.
19. Mainiero MB, Cinelli CM, Koelliker SL, Graves TA, Chung MA. Axillary ultrasound and fine-needle aspiration in the preoperative evaluation of the breast cancer patient: an algorithm based on tumor size and lymph node appearance. AJR Am J Roentgenol. 2010;195(5):1261–7.

Chapter 5
Abdominal Imaging

Surabhi Bajpai and Dushyant Sahani

Introduction

Diseases of the abdomen and pelvis can have a bewildering array of clinical presentations as a result of pathological conditions involving either the gastrointestinal (GI) or the genitourinary (GU) system. The diagnosis and management of these patients therefore is often clinically challenging and can represent an enigma despite or perhaps even due to the availability of numerous laboratory investigations. The introduction of imaging has opened new methods to evaluate patients presenting with diseases of the abdomen and pelvis. Imaging provides a unique inside view of the abdomen, and it frequently aids a treating physician in unraveling its complex mysteries. The explosion of various imaging modalities over the past century, ranging from plain radiography to magnetic resonance imaging (MRI), has revolutionized diagnosis and follow-up of patients with various types of pathology in the abdomen and pelvis. Continued advancements in the past few decades, particularly in cross-sectional imaging modalities such as multidetector computed tomography (MDCT) and MRI, have made imaging an integral tool in patient diagnosis and management. Indeed, an ultrasound (US) or CT scan is often among the initial investigations performed in a patient presenting to the emergency room with abdominal complaints. Despite their immense benefits, judicious use of imaging techniques is imperative, not only to avoid excessive economic burden on our healthcare system, but also to prevent unnecessary exposure to ionizing radiation with techniques such as fluoroscopy or CT scans (Table 5.1). In this chapter, our aim is to provide an overview of the various imaging techniques available in the interrogation of patients with signs and symptoms related to the abdomen and pelvis.

S. Bajpai, D.M.R.D. • D. Sahani, M.D. (✉)
Department of Radiology, Division of Abdominal Imaging and Intervention, Massachusetts General Hospital, Harvard Medical School, 55 Fruit Street, Boston, MA 02114, USA
e-mail: dsahani@partners.org

W.R. Reinus (ed.), *Clinician's Guide to Diagnostic Imaging*,
DOI 10.1007/978-1-4614-8769-2_5, © Springer Science+Business Media New York 2014

Table 5.1 Imaging modalities for the evaluation of abdominal pathology

Imaging modality	Indications and advantages	Limitations
Abdominal radiographs (KUB, obstructive series)	To demonstrate free air, bowel obstruction, calculi/calcification, foreign body, soft tissue mass displacing the bowel loops, ancillary findings like bone involvement	– Has a low sensitivity and specificity – Poor anatomic localization
Fluoroscopy	To demonstrate bowel motility, strictures, gastric reflux, gastric emptying In post op cases to demonstrate anastomotic leaks	
US	– Noninvasive and portable	– Subjective and operator-dependent
	– No radiation	– Decreased accuracy in patients with large body habitus
	– First imaging modality for • Right upper quadrant • Female pelvis • Pediatric patients	– Low sensitivity and specificity
CT	– High resolution	– Exposure to ionizing radiation
	– Wide coverage – Rapid investigation	– Limited application in patients with contrast allergies or abnormal renal function
	– 24/7 Access	
MRI	– Focused examination – Ideal for biliary/common bile duct evaluation – Imaging of choice for extended evaluation of pelvic pathology in women – Useful in pregnant patients – Monitoring of young patients with Crohn's disease to avoid excessive radiation	– Limited availability – Cost – Claustrophobia

Imaging Techniques: Overview

Plain Radiography/Fluoroscopy

Imaging evaluation of patients presenting with clinical signs and symptoms localizing to the diseases of the abdomen often begins with an abdominal radiograph or kidney–ureter–bladder (KUB) radiograph or an obstructive series of radiographs (usually consisting of either erect and supine or lateral decubitus and supine abdomen images). Plain radiography is an inexpensive imaging technique that is performed in patients with findings of an acute abdomen for the diagnosis of bowel obstruction, bowel perforation, or urinary stones. Plain radiographs also contribute to the routine care of patients to confirm the position of various tubes (nasogastric tube or drainage catheters) and as follow-up examinations in patients with ileus. Plain film radiography can be done rapidly and portably, allowing detection of several acute abdominal emergencies such as perforated viscus or bowel obstruction. Its disadvantages include lack of contrast resolution and an inability to differentiate various intra-abdominal structures.

Fluoroscopic imaging techniques performed after instillation of oral contrast agents is a great tool to evaluate diseases of both the GI and GU tracts. It is a dynamic imaging technique that is particularly valuable in detection of abnormalities affecting bowel motility. This includes evaluation of esophageal motility disorders in patients with dysphagia, heart burn, or chest pain. Fluoroscopic imaging with oral contrast is especially valuable in postoperative patients to assess the integrity of the gastrointestinal tract after bowel anastomotic surgery. Early identification of anastomotic leaks in the postoperative period allows a surgeon to plan appropriate early interventions. Conventional barium studies also can be used as first-line noninvasive diagnostic studies in patients with dyspepsia, weight loss, an abdominal mass, and partial obstruction. Double contrast techniques can provide good detail of the bowel mucosa allowing identification of ulcerations, small protrusions, and any strictures.

Ultrasound

Ultrasound (US) is a valuable noninvasive imaging technique that uses sound waves to create images of internal structures. This imaging technique does not expose the patient to ionizing radiation and is performed by placing an US probe (a transducer) onto the skin over the organ of interest. US provides real time gray scale images of various structures within the abdomen, including deeper organs. This imaging technique is routinely used to evaluate the gallbladder, liver, bile ducts, spleen, pancreas, kidneys, uterus, ovaries, and abdominal cavity.

The main advantages of US include:

1. US is universally available, easy to use, and is easily performed portably at the patient's bedside.
2. The real time, dynamic nature of US allows evaluation of motion in real time, e.g., to monitor peristalsis, observe fetal movements in pregnant women, and examine the effects of maneuvers, e.g., Valsalva and Mueller maneuvers, and gravity on internal organs.
3. The real time nature of US permits analysis of effects of graded compression on various structures to help determine tissue stiffness, i.e., rigid vs. soft. This use is not limited to the abdomen and in fact is a mainstay in evaluation of deep venous thrombosis in the limbs.
4. It allows direct visualization of blood flow and pulsations within vessels and masses.
5. US is an excellent tool to perform image guided interventional procedures.

US is suitable for both focused examination and for routine screening. As a screening tool, US is frequently used in the diagnosis of an obvious abdominal mass, peritoneal fluid collections such as ascites, and in the evaluation of hydrobilia or hydronephrosis. It is often performed as an initial imaging study for the evaluation of abdominal pain particularly in patients with right upper quadrant pain as it allows accurate diagnosis of acute cholecystitis. US plays an equally critical role in evaluation of lower abdominal pain and bleeding in women of childbearing age. In addition to allowing the detection of various conditions, US is a safe technique to guide aspiration and drainage of fluid collections/abscesses to determine their nature.

Recent advances in US include harmonic imaging, 3-dimensional (3-D) imaging, and sono-elastography [1, 2]. Harmonic imaging uses ultrasonic sound waves similar to US, but requires a broad transducer bandwidth. Harmonic imaging is superior to conventional US as it provides better lesion visibility, improves diagnostic confidence, and typically shows enhanced contrast by removing image noise. Harmonic imaging is generally useful for depicting cystic lesions, deep seated vascular structures, and those lesions containing echogenic tissues such as fat, calcium, or air.

3D volumetric sonography allows 3D reconstructions of anatomic structures from US images. It has shown great benefit in fetal ultrasonography because it permits easy identification of fetal anatomy and confident interpretation of congenital anomalies [1, 2]. 3D imaging is also routinely used to evaluate uterine abnormalities including depiction of congenital uterine anomalies and visualization of the position of intrauterine contraceptive devices. 3D imaging increases the confidence of needle placement during interventional procedures because it shows three planes simultaneously.

Despite these advantages, caution should be used when utilizing US for investigation. Obesity, the presence of dense overlying tissue and gaseous distention, can degrade US images because high frequency sound waves do not penetrate these tissues well. Poor penetration can limit the technical utility of abdominal ultrasound or even render it completely unable to visualize target organs. US is also operator-dependent, relying greatly on the skills and experience of the sonographer. Incorrectly performed scans can create a level of uncertainty in the interpretation of images and the diagnosis of pathology. Because of the comparatively narrow field of view produced by current transducers and the freehand method with which scans are performed, it is even possible to overlook pathology in some circumstances. Some have likened US to looking through a keyhole. Therefore it is of utmost importance to be sure the sonographer is well-trained and experienced. Of course, radiologists ultimately interpret the studies.

Multidetector CT

The advent of multidetector CT (MDCT) has provided impressive diagnostic benefits in the management of abdominal and pelvic disorders [3]. Utilization of MDCT scans in patients presenting with abdominal pain has undergone explosive growth.

Today, over 20 % of patients presenting to an emergency department with abdominal complaints undergo a CT examination. This represents a nearly tenfold increase in CT utilization over a 12-year period [4]. The high contrast resolution of CT makes it the preferred modality for high accuracy evaluation of both solid and hollow visceral pathology in the abdomen and pelvis.

The main advantages of MDCT include:

1. MDCT is universally available and easily accessible (24 hrs a day, 7 days a week).
2. MDCT allows rapid image acquisition with an ability to scan multiple body parts at the same time.
3. Standardized scanning protocols and image display patterns make interpretation easier.
4. It can be used for screening as well as for focused problem solving.
5. Its value can be augmented by administering oral and intravenous contrast, depending on the application.
6. CT has the capability to obtain images rapidly in sequences through a volume of tissue. This capability allows CT to depict different phases of filling of the vascular system as in CT angiography.

Despite these benefits, one of the major drawbacks of CT imaging is exposure to ionizing radiation, raising concerns about its long-term mutagenic and carcinogenic effects particularly in young patients who undergo multiple CT examinations [5]. The radiation dose is often dependent on type of examination with increased exposure encountered in CT exams with multiple phases such as arterial, venous and delayed phase.

In order to answer many clinical questions, CT of the abdomen and pelvis requires injection of intravenous iodinated contrast material (IVCM). Contrast enhanced MDCT studies improve lesion detection and characterization and also allow differentiation of lymph nodes from vascular structures. On the other hand, non-contrast CT, i.e., without intravenous contrast, is often sufficient to diagnose urinary tract stones and to identify suspected intra-abdominal hematomas.

For most applications, oral contrast material (OCM) also is administered routinely prior to a CT of the abdomen and pelvis. Intraluminal oral contrast is essential to help differentiate abnormal mesenteric lymph nodes from unopacified bowel loops, to facilitate detection of bowel abnormalities, to identify bowel perforations or anastomotic leaks, and to distinguish bowel from some extra intestinal pathology such as abscesses.

The OCM chosen for a given application can be positive or negative/neutral as indicated by its density measurements on the scan. Positive OCM includes dilute liquid barium suspensions and water-soluble iodine solutions, e.g., Gastrograffin, both of which appear denser than water on the scan. Negative/neutral OCM includes water and low-density barium solutions such as Volumen. Positive OCM is adequate for most indications in the abdomen, but neutral OCM is preferred for dedicated examinations that target the bowel itself, i.e., CT enterography (CTE). Iodinated contrast also can be injected through a catheter into the urinary bladder to diagnose urinary bladder rupture in patients with pelvic trauma, i.e., CT cystography (Table 5.2).

Table 5.2 MDCT protocols for imaging of the abdomen and pelvis

MDCT protocols	Clinical indications	Additional points
No oral contrast	High grade small bowel obstruction, unstable patients, CT angiographic studies, and suspected gastrointestinal bleed	Oral contrast can interfere with 3D imaging
Rectal contrast	Appendicitis, diverticulitis	
Intravenous contrast agent	Used in all indications except in most cases of ureteral stones/flank pain	Intravenous contrast agent opacifies the abdominal vasculature and provides useful information regarding the enhancement patterns of parenchymal organs and intestine Intravenous contrast can be given in doubtful cases of ureteral stones
Faster injection rate of intravenous contrast	GI bleed/bowel ischemia/hemorrhage/ vascular complications	
Dual phase (arterial and venous)	Liver or pancreatic mass	
Delayed phase	Hematuria and pelvic pathology	

Magnetic Resonance Imaging

Typically, MRI of the abdomen and pelvis is reserved for problem solving, usually as a targeted study with a specific question in mind. It is also the investigation of choice in patients with a history of allergy to iodinated contrast who, as a consequence, cannot undergo a contrast enhanced MDCT. MRI does have drawbacks since it is expensive relative to other diagnostic imaging examinations, and even with today's wider and shorter bore scanners, claustrophobic patients may be unable to tolerate being in the bore of the scanner. In addition, the long scanning times required to complete a study make MRI undesirable for acutely ill patients and for patients who are unable to lie still during image acquisition.

The superior contrast and soft tissue resolution of MRI makes it an invaluable technique in visualization of the hepato-pancreato-biliary pathology. The enhanced contrast resolution of MR coupled with its ability to depict tissues using multiple sequences to accentuate different tissue parameters have elevated MR as the preferred imaging modality for characterization of hepatic lesions. For example, MR is excellent at detecting early hepatocellular carcinomas in patients with chronic parenchymal liver disease such as that resulting from Hepatitis B or C infections.

Furthermore, the recent availability of specific hepatobiliary contrast agents has improved MR's detection of hepatic metastases. MR plays a crucial role in monitoring the response of known hepatic malignancies to systemic chemotherapy, trans-arterial chemo embolization (TACE), and percutaneous ablative therapies, e.g., radiofrequency ablation (RFA). MR is considered very accurate in assessment of pancreatic lesions, particularly cystic lesions, and to evaluate the pancreatic duct. Magnetic resonance cholangiopancreatography (MRCP) provides two dimensional (2D) and 3D views of the biliary tree and pancreatic ducts and so in many cases has supplanted standard ERCP for noninvasive evaluation of the biliary tree.

MR enterography (MRE), also called MR enteroclysis, is a focused MR examination dedicated to evaluation of small bowel pathology. It has gained acceptance in the past decade as a replacement to MDCT because of concerns about high radiation exposure from repeated MDCT studies in patients with inflammatory bowel disease. MRE provides exquisite detail of small bowel pathology and is accurate in the identification of extra intestinal complications such as abscess and fistula.

MRI precisely depicts uterine and adnexal pathology and so is integral to staging of uterine and ovarian malignancies. In addition, because MRI does not employ ionizing radiation, it can be used repeatedly in young individuals and in pregnant women without fear of carcinogenesis. MR is performed routinely for local staging of patients with prostate and rectal cancer, both before surgery and afterwards to monitor therapeutic response.

Imaging for Abdominal pain

Abdominal pain is a common presentation and often the most challenging complaint to evaluate [5, 6]. This symptom accounts for nearly 2 % of outpatient visits and nearly 5 % of patients presenting to the emergency department. Most often the etiology of the pain is benign, but nearly 10 % of patients who present to the emergency department with abdominal pain have a life-threatening problem that often requires surgery (Fig. 5.1).

Evaluation of these patients requires a thorough and logical approach that depends on the location of the pain. For example, in conditions such as acute appendicitis or cholecystitis accurate pain localization has very strong predictive value [5]. Although imaging is often the final arbiter in the patient's evaluation, it should not be considered as a substitute for a careful history and physical examination along with relevant laboratory tests (Tables 5.3 and 5.4). Imaging techniques such as plain radiographs or ultrasound should be considered as first-line tools before opting for advanced techniques such as CT or MRI [5, 6].

Right Upper Quadrant Pain

Although the most common cause of right upper quadrant pain is acute cholecystitis, the spectrum of diseases that manifest as acute right upper quadrant pain also includes complications from cholecystitis, choledocholithiasis, biliary colic caused by hemobilia, ascending cholangitis, liver abscess, recurrent pyogenic cholangiohepatitis, gallbladder torsion, hepatic artery aneurysm, and complications of liver masses, such as rupture and hemorrhage [6–9].

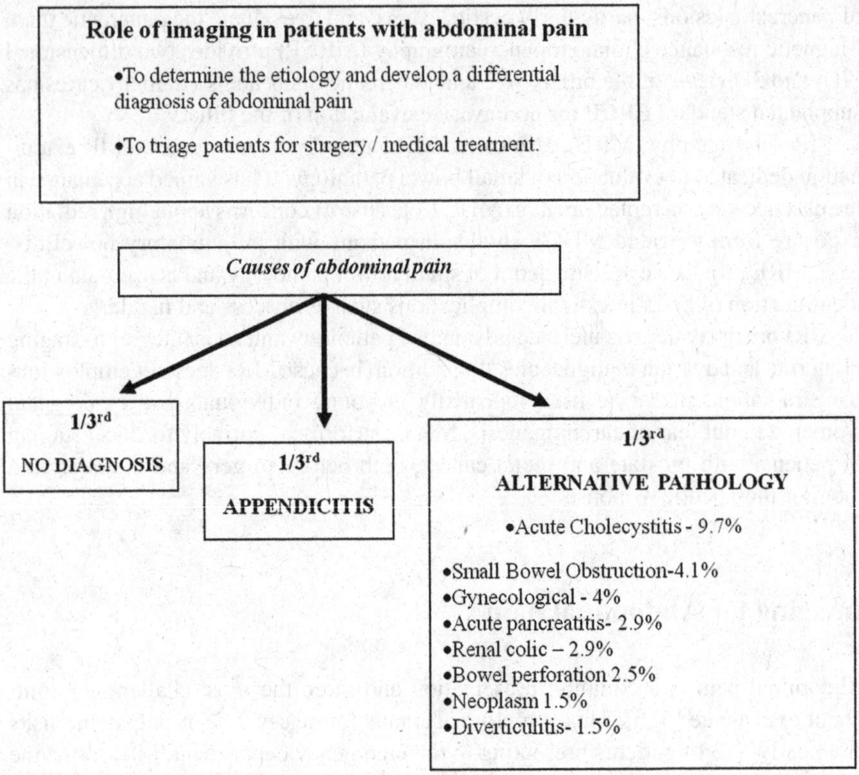

Fig. 5.1 Flow chart demonstrating the role of imaging in patients with abdominal pain [18, 19]

US is the primary imaging modality used to evaluate acute right upper quadrant pain (Fig. 5.2). It is highly sensitive and specific for the detection of gallstones and biliary dilatation. The accuracy of US (88 %) in patients with suspected acute cholecystitis is similar to that of scintigraphy (85 %). As a result, US, because it is less time-consuming than scintigraphy and uses no ionizing radiation, has replaced scintigraphy as the preferred exam for these patients [7–9]. Not only does US more easily demonstrate complications of acute cholecystitis than scintigraphy, e.g., gangrenous and emphysematous change, but it also may reveal an alternate diagnosis as the cause of the patient's symptoms.

US is superior to MDCT as the initial imaging technique for assessment of acute right upper quadrant pain caused by biliary disease, because ultrasound allows evaluation of a sonographic Murphy's sign, pain elicited by direct pressure on the abdomen with the transducer placed over the gallbladder. This is sensitive for diagnosis of acute cholecystitis [8, 9]. In addition, gallstones can be better detected on US than MDCT. Moreover, US is rapid, easily accessible, and portable. As mentioned above, US's usefulness is limited in obese patients because the US beam poorly penetrates adipose tissue, and this results in poor image quality and anatomic detail.

Table 5.3 Various causes and imaging investigation of choice in abdominal pain

Symptom	Causes	Imaging modality of choice	Second most preferred modality	Other imaging modalities
Right upper quadrant	Biliary: cholecystitis, cholelithiasis, cholangitis Colonic: colitis, diverticulitis Hepatic: abscess, hepatitis, mass Renal: nephrolithiasis, pyelonephritis	Ultrasound	MDCT	MRI—biliary anomalies HIDA—functional evaluation of hepatobiliary system
Epigastric pain	Biliary: cholecystitis, cholelithiasis, cholangitis Gastric: esophagitis, gastritis, peptic ulcer Pancreatic: mass, pancreatitis	Ultrasound	MDCT	
Left upper quadrant	Gastric: esophagitis, gastritis, peptic ulcer Pancreatic: mass, pancreatitis Renal: nephrolithiasis, pyelonephritis	MDCT	Ultrasound	
Right lower quadrant	Colonic: appendicitis, colitis, diverticulitis, IBD, IBS Gynecologic: ectopic pregnancy, fibroids, ovarian mass, torsion, PID Renal: nephrolithiasis, pyelonephritis	MDCT (transvaginal sonography*)	Ultrasound	
Left lower quadrant	Colonic: colitis, diverticulitis, IBD, IBS Gynecologic: ectopic pregnancy, fibroids, ovarian mass, torsion, PID Renal: nephrolithiasis, pyelonephritis	MDCT (transvaginal sonography*)	Ultrasound	
Diffuse pain with rigid abdomen	Bowel perforation	Abdominal radiograph	MDCT	
Abdominal distension	Small bowel obstruction	Obstructive series	MDCT	Fluoroscopy in partial obstruction

*Transvaginal ultrasound is the imaging investigation of choice in women of childbearing age

Table 5.4 Imaging investigations in specific abdominal conditions

Diagnosis	Imaging modality for initial evaluation	Role of other imaging modalities	Additional points
Acute pancreatitis	MDCT	MRI to evaluate pancreatic duct disruption/structural anomalies	
Acute cholecystitis	US	MDCT in equivocal cases Cholescintigraphy	
Choledocholitiasis	US or MDCT	MRCP or ERCP	
Acute appendicitis	MDCT	MRI in pregnant patients US in thin and young patients US in pediatric patients	
Adnexal torsion	US with Doppler	MRI in patients with large body habitus and when ovary is not visible because of intervening structures	Doppler may still demonstrate flow despite ovarian torsion due to secondary blood supply by uterine artery branches
Pelvic inflammatory disease	US MDCT—with more diffuse symptoms	MRI in equivocal cases as it depicts adnexal edema	

Table 5.5 Bile duct obstruction: accuracy of various imaging modalities

Imaging modalities	Accuracy for common bile duct stones (%)	Limitations
US	25–55	Operator-dependent, limited visibility due to bowel gas
CT	80–90	Radiation exposure and limited visualization of non-calcified stones
MRI	67–100	Not easily available, expensive, and long scanning times.
ERCP/Endoscopic Ultrasound (EUS)	80–100	Invasive, operator-dependent, and limited field of view

MDCT is often an excellent alternative to US in evaluation of right upper quadrant pain for some patients. It is superior to US in determining the cause and the extent of disease in situations where visibility with US is limited (e.g., open wounds, surgical dressings, and obesity). MDCT also is valuable in the assessment of complications of acute cholecystitis and in patients with abdominal pain after cholecystectomy.

On the other hand, the accuracy of MDCT is limited in patients with common bile duct stones and in cases with complicated ductal anatomy. In these cases MRI, with its excellent soft tissue contrast, and MRCP provide detailed diagnostic information about the biliary tree (Table 5.5). The recent development of fast MR

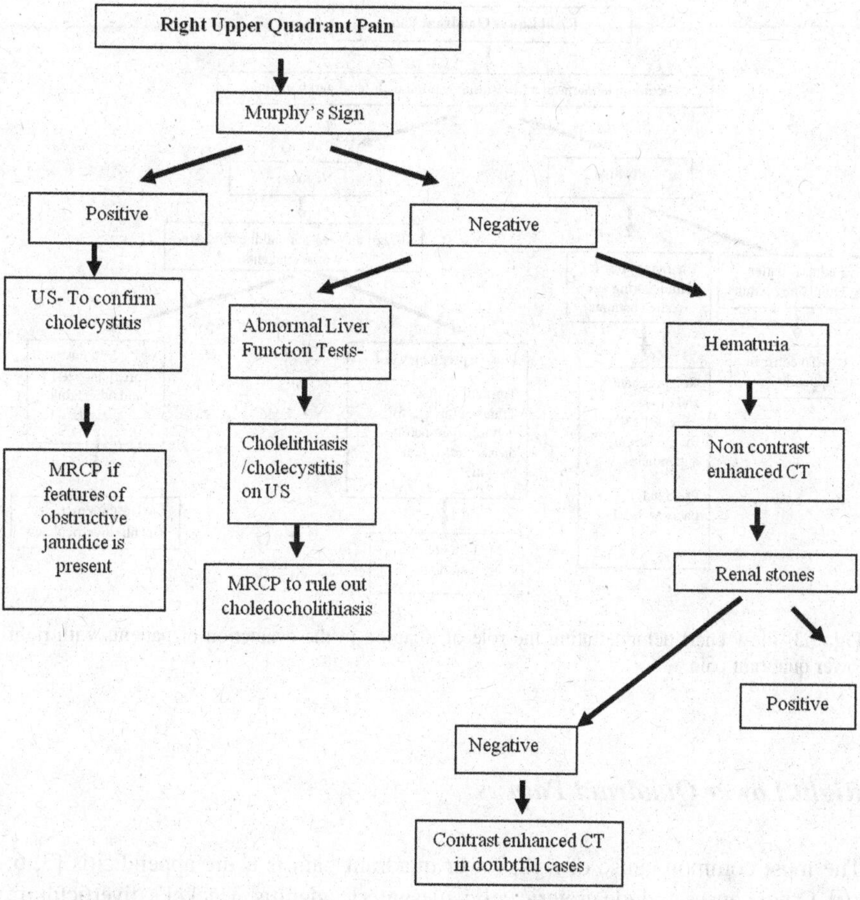

Fig. 5.2 Flow chart demonstrating the role of imaging in the evaluation of patients with right upper quadrant pain

techniques has reduced imaging time, and thus MR can be performed in emergency situations. Almost 15–30 % of patients with acute biliary disorders require MRI. MRCP, because it uses no ionizing radiation, also plays an important role in evaluation of pregnant patients with acute pancreatobiliary disease. Endoscopic retrograde cholangiopancreatography (ERCP) with papillotomy is the preferred next step in the management of patients shown to have choledocholithiasis and biliary dilatation on US, CT, or MR.

Despite US's hegemony, cholescintigraphy remains an important noninvasive test to diagnose acute cholecystitis because it can directly show cystic duct obstruction. Failure of gall bladder filling with radiotracer in the presence of normal hepatic uptake and biliary excretion indicates acute cholecystitis whereas normal gall bladder visualization excludes the diagnosis.

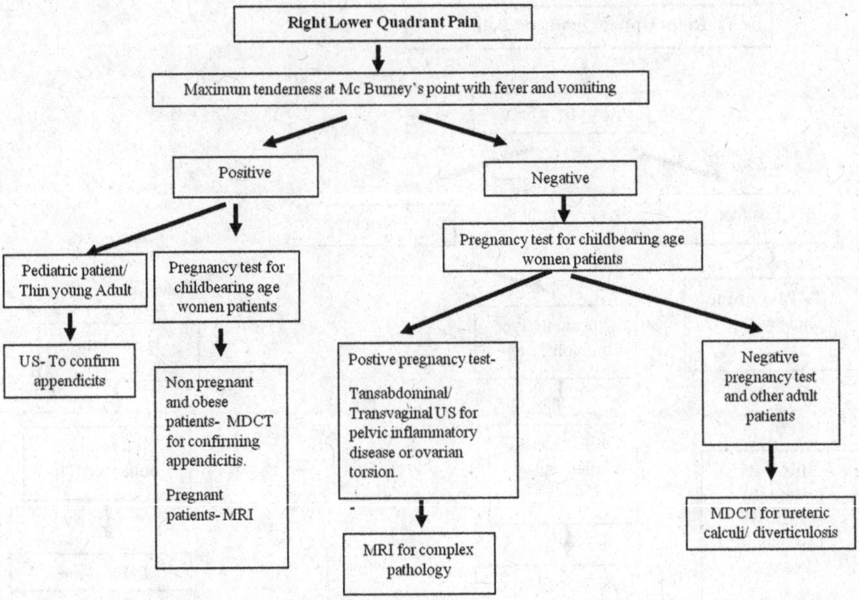

Fig. 5.3 Flow chart demonstrating the role of imaging in the evaluation of patients with right lower quadrant pain

Right Lower Quadrant Pain

The most common cause of right lower quadrant pain is acute appendicitis [3, 6, 10]. Other causes include ureteric colic, mesenteric adenitis, Meckel's diverticulum, and occasionally right-sided diverticulitis (Fig. 5.3). In an immunocompromised patient typhilitis (cecal inflammation from any number of etiologies) is a common cause. In women of childbearing age, ovarian torsion, tubo-ovarian abscess, and pelvic inflammatory disease should also be considered [3, 6, 10].

MDCT has proven itself as the most accurate study for evaluating patients where the clinical diagnosis of acute appendicitis is uncertain. Routine creation of multiplanar reformations compliments axial images and improves reader confidence in the diagnosis. MDCT is also valuable to exclude other causes of right lower quadrant pain such as ureteric calculi, right-sided diverticulitis, and pelvic pathology.

Trans-abdominal and transvaginal sonography are preferred over MDCT in the initial evaluation of women of childbearing age with right lower quadrant pain. Transvaginal sonography is accurate in the detection of various causes of pelvic pathology, including ovarian mass, ovarian torsion, and tubo-ovarian abscess. In those patients in whom sonographic examination reveals complex pathology, MRI of the pelvis is an appropriate next step as a problem-solving tool.

Left Upper Quadrant Pain

The most common causes of left upper quadrant (LUQ) pain are splenic pathology with or without splenomegaly and renal stones [5, 6]. Other causes include esophagitis, gastritis, pancreatic, and renal pathology aside from stones. Rarely, elderly patients may develop mesenteric ischemia, which can lead to ischemic colitis. This typically presents with LUQ pain and hematochezia. Ischemic colitis typically arises in the region of the splenic flexure because of the relatively poor blood supply in the watershed between the middle colic and left colic arteries.

Either US or MDCT could be chosen as the initial investigation of LUQ pain depending on the patient's symptoms. MDCT is more accurate than US in detecting causes of LUQ pain, especially in the detection of urinary tract stones. CT is also beneficial in defining extent of abnormality in diseases such as pancreatitis, splenic abscess, and ischemic colitis. On the other hand, US is less expensive than CT and uses no ionizing radiation. As a result, US reasonably may be considered as an initial examination in the evaluation of LUQ pain.

Left Lower Quadrant Pain

The most common cause of left lower quadrant (LLQ) pain in adults is acute diverticulitis [6, 11]. Other differential considerations include urinary tract stones and, in women, gynecological pathology. MDCT is the imaging investigation of choice in patients with left lower quadrant pain. It not only allows confident diagnosis of diverticulitis but also accurately diagnoses renal and ureteral stones. Excluding gynecologic disease, the main role of imaging in LLQ pain is to diagnose or exclude diverticulitis, and if present, to evaluate the extent of disease and to detect complications such as abscess formation.

In the past, contrast enema was the primary investigation performed to diagnose diverticulitis. Although barium or water-soluble contrast enema have high sensitivity for the diagnosis of sigmoid diverticulitis and other diseases such as ischemic colitis and inflammatory bowel disease, it is insensitive for detection of extramural processes that can mimic diverticulitis clinically. Thus, MDCT has supplanted contrast enema as the initial imaging test in patients with LLQ pain. In addition, because MDCT can identify the presence and extent of extramural complications of diverticulitis such as abscess, it facilitates the selection of medical or surgical therapy in this disease. MDCT also can be used to guide percutaneous drainage of abdominal abscesses and so eliminate the need for surgery.

Women of child bearing age with left lower quadrant pain should have a pelvic US as their initial investigation because of the frequency with which pain in this part of the abdomen arises from gynecologic abnormalities. Transvaginal ultrasound holds great importance in this setting as it can diagnose important causes of pain such as ectopic pregnancy and pelvic inflammatory disease. The particular imaging

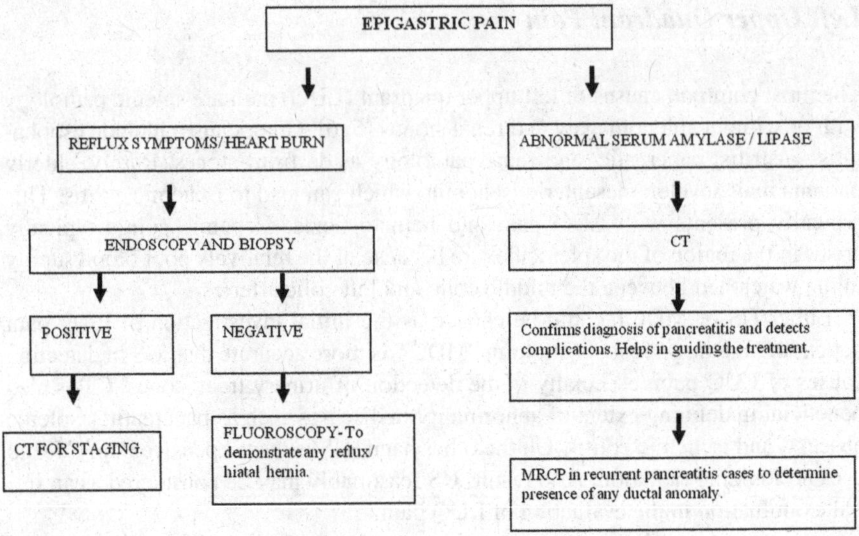

Fig. 5.4 Flow chart demonstrating the role of imaging in the evaluation of patients with epigastric pain

modality selected as an initial examination in these circumstances is usually based on the patient's age, gender, presenting symptoms, and laboratory results such as urine or serum human β-chorionic gonadatropin (βhCG) levels.

Epigastric Pain

The most common etiologies of epigastric pain arise from lower esophageal and/or gastric pathology (Fig. 5.4). Other causes include cholecystitis and pancreatitis. Rarely, a ventral epigastric hernia can present with epigastric pain. Endoscopy is the gold standard for detection of mucosal lesions of the esophagus and stomach and so is the initial test of choice. If endoscopy is negative and the patient's amylase and lipase are elevated, MDCT can confirm the diagnosis of pancreatitis as well as diagnose less common causes of pancreatitis besides alcohol ingestion such as biliary tract disease. CT is not only accurate in diagnosing early pancreatitis and defining the presence and extent of pancreatic and peri-pancreatic inflammation, but it also is accurate at identifying complications of pancreatitis such as pseudocyst and pancreatic necrosis.

Although most pancreatic pathology typically presents with symptoms other than pain, MDCT is accurate in detection and characterization of pancreatic masses including epithelial carcinoma. MR with MRCP, on the other hand, is superior to MDCT for characterization of subtle abnormalities including detection of mural nodules in pancreatic cysts and defining pancreatic ductal abnormalities. MRCP is of particular value in showing communication between cystic pancreatic lesions and the main pancreatic duct.

Imaging in Hepatobiliary Disorders

Imaging plays a crucial role in the evaluation of patients with symptoms related to hepatobiliary disorders. Jaundice and elevated transaminases are among the most common presenting symptoms in patients with hepatobiliary disease. Transabdominal US is the initial investigation of choice for these patients. In addition to visualizing the biliary tree, US can assess parenchymal diseases of the liver, including fatty infiltration and cirrhosis. In patients with cirrhosis, US is often chosen as a screening tool to detect focal lesions that might represent hepatocellular carcinoma. Complete imaging evaluation of liver lesions detected by ultrasound requires dynamic three-phase imaging with MDCT and MRI.

Imaging often plays a crucial role in identifying the cause of obstructive jaundice. Again, US is the initial imaging investigation for jaundiced patients and permits detection of intrahepatic and extrahepatic biliary duct dilatation. Both MDCT and MR are accurate at diagnosing the etiology of biliary obstruction, including choledocholithiasis and neoplastic lesions of the biliary ducts, pancreatic head, and periampullary region (Table 5.5). As a result, MDCT or MR with MRCP is usually chosen as the next study in the evaluation of the biliary tree pathology.

Hepatobiliary scintigraphy is more sensitive than US to diagnose low grade or early biliary obstruction. As a result, scintigraphy may be chosen as a first-line examination for suspected biliary obstruction or as a follow-on examination when US is negative but clinical suspicion persists. Another important role of hepatobiliary scintigraphy is in patients suspected of having a bile leak following cholecystectomy and biliary surgery. Hepatobiliary scintigraphy is more sensitive than US or CT for detection of biliary leaks. While CT and US may demonstrate the presence of fluid collection, scintigraphy is able to establish an active biliary leak as a etiology of the fluid collection.

Imaging of Bowel Abnormalities

Stomach and Duodenum

Optical endoscopy is the preferred investigation for evaluation of gastric and duodenal pathology as well as diseases of the colon. Imaging studies, particularly barium swallow and upper gastrointestinal studies, are still performed in patients with nonspecific symptoms related to the stomach and duodenum. Barium studies are useful also to define esophageal and gastric anatomy prior to bariatric surgery. Following gastrointestinal surgery, fluoroscopic studies with water-soluble contrast often are performed for depiction of integrity of the anastomosed segments, i.e., to detect anastomotic leaks and to identify causes of postoperative obstruction.

Small Bowel

Small bowel pathology always presents a diagnostic challenge to the gastroenterologist. Traditionally barium evaluation of the small bowel has been the standard diagnostic test. With the increasing use of MDCT for diagnosis of bowel abnormalities, however, fluoroscopic barium studies are waning. The utility of MDCT in small bowel diseases has increased further with the introduction of CT enterography (CTE), a dedicated CT examination of the bowel performed after ingestion of neutral oral contrast medium (OCM). MDCT has several advantages over fluoroscopic studies because in addition to depiction of luminal abnormalities, CT allows display of the entire intestinal wall thickness, its surrounding mesentery, and perienteric fat. CTE, with neutral OCM, permits excellent assessment of inflammatory and vascular disorders of the bowel. In addition, CT aids in the assessment of solid organs and so provides a global overview of the abdomen.

Thus, CTE has emerged as the first-line modality in the evaluation of suspected inflammatory bowel disease including Crohn's disease. It is used not only for diagnosis but also to monitor the course of the disease, including the effectiveness of therapy and detection of later complications such as abscess, fistula, and small bowel obstruction. As mentioned previously, MR enterography is gaining on CTE as an alternative to CT because of the hazards from repeated radiation exposure, particularly for follow-up examinations in patients with known disease.

Colon

Optical colonoscopy is considered the gold standard for evaluation of colonic disorders. Nonetheless, CT has a crucial role in diagnosis and management of both inflammatory and neoplastic diseases of the colon. MDCT is the primary imaging tool to stage patients with colon cancer as it provides detailed information on local tumor extension, lymph node involvement, and distant metastases, particularly to the liver. CT colonography provides virtual endoluminal visualization of the colon using 3D reconstruction techniques. This modality serves as an adjunct to screening optical colonoscopy in patients where optical colonoscopy is incomplete because of difficult anatomy, obstructing tumor, or diverticulosis. CT colonography offers complete evaluation of both luminal and extra-luminal abnormalities of the colon.

Its relative disadvantage to optical colonoscopy is the inability to biopsy lesions at the time of the examination. Thus, optical colonoscopy may be required after a positive CT colonoscopy. Depending upon the work flow in a hospital, this may require a second bowel preparation. Another indication for CT in colonic disease is in the evaluation of patients with colitis because CT clearly depicts the extent and severity of colonic involvement.

Gastrointestinal Bleeding

Gastrointestinal bleeding can occur due to a variety of pathologies affecting the bowel ranging from a tumor, ischemia to vascular malformations. Detection of the cause of the lesion aids in further management of the patient. While routine MDCT scan may aid in identifying malignant lesions, CT angiography can diagnose ischemic lesions and vascular malformations. Successful management of GI bleeding patients also depends on localization of bleeding site. While upper GI tract bleeding can be located with endoscopy and selective arteriography in the majority of cases, the lower GI bleeds, including the large and small bowels, are diagnosed most often with nuclear medicine studies. Scintigraphy studies have proven to be extremely sensitive with an ability to detect bleeds as low as 0.05–0.1 mL/min. Technetium^{99m} labeled red blood cell scintigraphy plays an important role in the evaluation of lower gastrointestinal bleeding owing to the limited sensitivity of endoscopy and intermittent bleeding. Radionuclide studies have typically been used as a screening examination to identify patients who require targeted angiography or surgery.

Hematuria

A wide variety of medical and surgical pathology, originating from any part of the urinary tract, can cause hematuria (Fig. 5.5). As a result it is a frequent indication for imaging of the urinary tract [12]. Hematuria is divided commonly into macroscopic hematuria or recurrent microscopic hematuria [12]. The risk of malignancy is higher in patients with macroscopic hematuria [12]. The incidence of malignancy is between10 and 28 % overall in cases of hematuria, and 10 % in patients younger than 40 years [12].

Radiologic investigation is performed after a complete clinical evaluation, urine analysis, and appropriate blood tests [13, 14]. In some circumstances imaging does not add value to a clinical diagnosis [13, 14], for example, in young women with clinical presentation of urinary tract infection, where hematuria completely resolves after successful therapy [12]. Similarly, patients with obvious evidence of glomerulonephropathy do not require an extensive imaging workup to rule out any surgical cause [12], but a baseline ultrasound evaluation is helpful in the morphological evaluation of the kidneys.

Combining imaging evaluation with optical cystoscopy, which has been proven to be most sensitive and accurate for detecting lesions in the urinary collecting system and urinary bladder, is the current practice to evaluate patients for surgical causes of hematuria [12]. Traditionally, prior to the development of MDCT, excretory urography was considered the standard in imaging of patients with hematuria [12]. Now, after performing standard contrast MDCT, obtaining thin section CT images after suitable delay provides visualization of the entire urinary tract because at this time the contrast agent completely opacifies the collecting system and the bladder. Patients scheduled for type of CT, known as CT

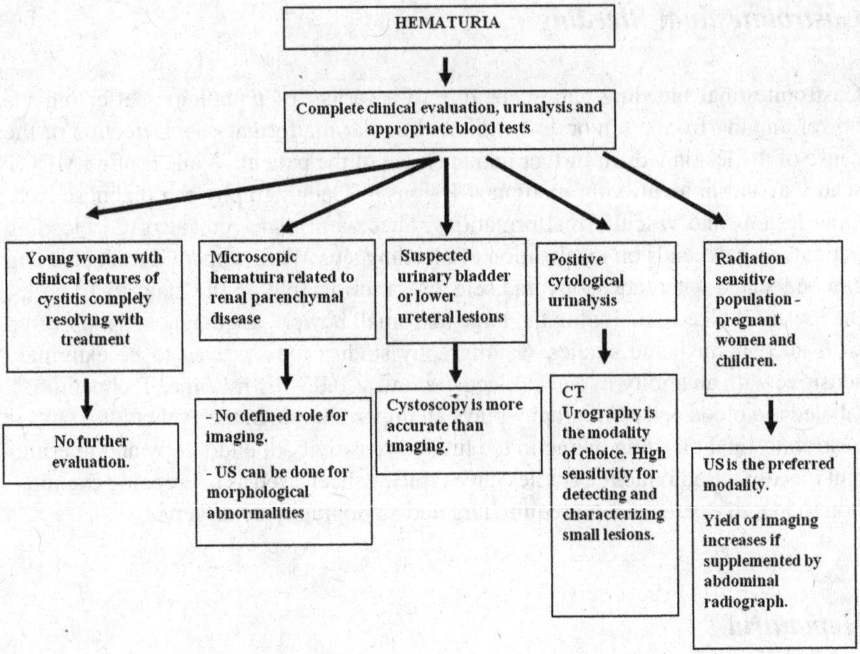

Fig. 5.5 Imaging algorithm for hematuria

urography, are hydrated prior to the CT examination and then given a low dose of diuretic at the time of the scan for optimal visualization of urinary tract [12]. CT Urography can detect the cause of hematuria with an overall sensitivity of 92–100 % and specificity of 89–97 % [12, 15]. It has now become the method of choice for hematuria, supplanting intravenous pyelography even though their appropriateness rating according to American College of Radiology (ACR) is the same [13, 14].

US is an appropriate first-line diagnostic test especially in children and pregnant women with hematuria, in whom ionizing radiation must be avoided [12–14]. US has low sensitivity for stone detection (19–32 %), but when pyelocalyceal dilatation is also present, the sensitivity is much better [12]. Because it has lower sensitivity relative to other cross-sectional imaging modalities, US also has a limited role in renal mass detection [13, 14]. On the other hand, it does play a role characterizing lesions identified on cross-sectional imaging, particularly determining whether they are cystic or solid and their degree of vascularity [13, 14]. US can reliably distinguish simple cysts, which are benign and require no follow-up, from less common complex masses demanding additional evaluation [13, 14].

MRI is an excellent technique to evaluate the renal parenchyma for masses and other abnormalities, but it is inferior to CT urography in diagnosing urothelial pathology at present [13, 14]. Thus, its role is mainly confined to patients who have a contraindication to intravenous iodinated contrast and in patients with concerns about the risks of radiation exposure [13, 14]. In addition, MRI is limited in patients with compromised renal function due to nephrogenic systemic fibrosis (NSS), which has been shown to be a potential complication of intravenous gadolinium contrast agents in patients with renal dysfunction [13, 14].

Adnexal Lesions and Female Pelvis

Ultrasound is the first-line imaging modality for evaluation of abnormalities of the female pelvis with high diagnostic accuracy for detecting both uterine and ovarian pathology [16]. US provides good morphologic detail and information about vascularity, thus helping to narrow the differential diagnosis, but it cannot always confidently differentiate malignant from benign masses [16]. Of course, findings on ultrasound must be correlated with the patient's clinical picture and laboratory tests, particularly pregnancy tests.

Sonographic evaluation of the female pelvis is performed both via trans-abdominal and transvaginal approaches. These techniques complement each other [16]. Transvaginal sonography (TVS) has improved resolution compared with the trans-abdominal (TAS) approach, permitting improved diagnostic confidence [16]. TVS allows better differentiation between cystic and solid masses adnexal lesions. TAS plays an important role in evaluating large pelvic masses which extend into the lower abdomen and helps define the mass' relationship with other pelvic structures [16]. Doppler US is useful to assess lesion vascularity and guide percutaneous procedures. As with all applications of US, the main limitations of pelvic US include a limited field of view and obscuration of pelvic organs by bowel gas and adipose tissue [16].

MRI plays a problem-solving role in the evaluation of pelvic pathology. It is being used increasingly because of its superior contrast resolution and the ability to provide good tissue characterization [16]. MRI is valuable in determining the origin of the mass (uterine versus ovarian versus non-gynecologic) and excluding malignancy in indeterminate adnexal masses [16]. It currently has an established role in diagnosis of adenomyosis, staging of pelvic malignancies, evaluation of uterine and Mullerian duct anomalies, and in presurgical workup for pelvic floor prolapse [16]. Since MR depicts the ovarian vascular pedicle well, it also plays a role in the emergency evaluation of ovarian torsion. Table 5.6 provides the imaging guidelines for clinical variants of adnexal lesions.

Acute Non-traumatic Scrotal Pain

The scrotum is mainly imaged for two clinical indications: incidentally discovered painless scrotal mass and an acutely painful scrotum which may be spontaneous or

Table 5.6 Imaging guidelines for adnexal lesions

Clinical condition	Imaging modality of choice	Second most preferred modality	Other imaging modality
Clinically suspected adnexal mass in nonpregnant young patient	US (all three tests TAS, TVS, and Doppler may be performed depending on the clinical condition)	MRI pelvis with or without contrast. Problem-solving tool if US is inconclusive	
Follow-up of a complex solid adnexal lesion in a young nonpregnant patient	US	MRI in cases where the lesion is very large and the origin is unclear	CT used for staging if origin of mass is non-gynecological
Follow-up of a persistent or enlarging solid or complex mass	MRI (if a conservative treatment is elected and malignancy cannot be excluded)	CT (staging of ovarian cancer or evaluation of primary tumor in case of suspected metastases)	
Nonpregnant young patient with a simple cyst >6 cm	US (to visualize the lesion and analyze the blood flow)	MRI (for large lesion with limited US findings)	Image-guided aspiration (may be helpful if infectious etiology is suspected. Can be used as a therapeutic tool)
Initial evaluation in a postmenopausal patient with suspected adnexal mass	US (all three tests TAS, TVS, and Doppler may be performed depending on the clinical condition)	MRI pelvis with or without contrast. Problem-solving tool if US is inconclusive	
Follow-up in a postmenopausal patient with a large >5 cm ovarian cyst	US (to visualize the lesion and analyze the blood flow)	MRI (for large lesion with limited US findings)	

the result of trauma [17]. Several imaging modalities are available for imaging the scrotum, but today US and MRI are used predominantly because they provide rapid and accurate diagnosis [17]. US, in conjunction with the contemporaneous physical examination, is the mainstay of imaging and often the only modality necessary [17]. MRI plays a problem-solving role when US findings are equivocal or suboptimal [17]. If US diagnoses a mass and malignancy is suspected, MDCT will be necessary to evaluate the possibility of metastatic disease. Table 5.7 provides a comparative analysis of the various modalities used in the imaging of scrotum.

Table 5.7 Imaging modalities for evaluation of acute scrotum

Imaging modality	Comments and advantages	Limitations
US	– Mainstay of imaging of scrotum – Always performed in conjunction with clinical examination – Provides high resolution images of scrotum and its contents – Relatively inexpensive and quick to perform – Color Doppler evaluation can assess for testicular perfusion – Allows dynamic maneuvers such as Valsalva maneuver to assess for varicocele – Allows evaluation of extra-testicular anatomy and pathologies in the spermatic cord and scrotal sac	– Operator skill-dependent – Detorsed testes may be missed on US – Torsion of testicular appendage, a common cause of testicular pain in children can be difficult to diagnose on US
MRI	– Can detect undescended testis not seen on US – Provides excellent tissue details – Contrast enhanced MR allows diagnosis of benign masses equivocal on US – Allows evaluation of retroperitoneal structures at the site of testicular lymphatic drainage – Allows evaluation of extra-testicular anatomy and pathologies in the spermatic cord and scrotal sac	– Relatively expensive – Motion sensitive and requires more time to perform the study – Cannot be used in patients with pacemakers, implants, and claustrophobia
Tc^{99m} Scintigraphy	– Allows reasonably accurate differentiation between testicular ischemia and infection in adults	– Infrequently used due to longer examination times, less availability, exposure to ionizing radiation, and limited diagnostic capabilities in young boys – Limited experience among trained personnel for performance and interpretation of these exams

Conclusion

Imaging plays a crucial role in the evaluation of patients presenting with symptoms related to the abdomen. Technologic advancements in the realm of imaging provides the referring physician with a wide range of imaging modalities to choose from in order to unravel simple and challenging cases. Appropriate use of existing imaging technology is imperative to provide better quality care to patients and to avoid both excess radiation exposure and an unwarranted use of healthcare resources.

References

1. Campani R, Bottinelli O, Calliada F, Coscia D. The latest in ultrasound: three-dimensional imaging. Part II. Eur J Radiol. 1998;27 Suppl 2:S183–7.
2. Harvey CJ, Pilcher JM, Eckersley RJ, Blomley MJ, Cosgrove DO. Advances in ultrasound. Clin Radiol. 2002;57:157–77.
3. Leschka S, Alkadhi H, Wildermuth S, Marincek B. Multi-detector computed tomography of acute abdomen. Eur Radiol. 2005;15:2435–47.
4. Kocher KE, Meurer WJ, Fazel R, Scott PA, Krumholz HM, Nallamothu BK. National trends in use of computed tomography in the emergency department. Ann Emerg Med. 2011;58: 452–62.
5. Cartwright SL, Knudson MP. Evaluation of acute abdominal pain in adults. Am Fam Physician. 2008;77:971–8.
6. Shuman WP, Ralls PW, Balfe DM, et al. Imaging evaluation of patients with acute abdominal pain and fever. American College of Radiology. ACR Appropriateness Criteria. Radiology. 2000;215(Suppl):209–12.
7. Bree RL, Ralls PW, Balfe DM, et al. Evaluation of patients with acute right upper quadrant pain. American College of Radiology. ACR Appropriateness Criteria. Radiology. 2000; 215(Suppl):153–7.
8. Hanbidge AE, Buckler PM, O'Malley ME, Wilson SR. From the RSNA refresher courses: imaging evaluation for acute pain in the right upper quadrant. Radiographics. 2004;24: 1117–35.
9. Spence SC, Teichgraeber D, Chandrasekhar C. Emergent right upper quadrant sonography. J Ultrasound Med. 2009;28:479–96.
10. Ralls PW, Balfe DM, Bree RL, et al. Evaluation of acute right lower quadrant pain. American College of Radiology. ACR Appropriateness Criteria. Radiology. 2000;215(Suppl):159–66.
11. Hammond NA, Nikolaidis P, Miller FH. Left lower-quadrant pain: guidelines from the American College of Radiology appropriateness criteria. Am Fam Physician. 2010;82: 766–70.
12. van der Molen AJ, Hovius M. Hematuria: a problem-based imaging algorithm illustrating the recent Dutch guidelines on hematuria. AJR Am J Roentgenol. 2012;198(6):1256–65.
13. Newhouse JH, Amis Jr ES, Bigongiari LR, et al. Radiologic investigation of patients with hematuria. American College of Radiology. ACR Appropriateness Criteria. Radiology. 2000; 215(Suppl):687–91.
14. Royal SA, Slovis TL, Kushner DC, et al. Hematuria. American College of Radiology. ACR Appropriateness Criteria. Radiology. 2000;215(Suppl):841–6.
15. Lang EK, Thomas R, Davis R, et al. Multiphasic helical computerized tomography for the assessment of microscopic hematuria: a prospective study. J Urol. 2004;171:237–43.
16. Bohm-Velez M, Mendelson E, Bree R, et al. Suspected adnexal masses. American College of Radiology. ACR Appropriateness Criteria. Radiology. 2000;215(Suppl):931–8.
17. Asrani A, Morani AK, Colen RR. Imaging of scrotum. In: Sahani D, Samir A, editors. Abdominal imaging. 1st ed. Maryland, Missouri: Saunders Elsevier; 2010.
18. de Bombal F. Diagnosis of acute abdominal pain. Edinburgh: Churchill Livingstone; 1991.
19. Gore RM, Miller FH, Pereles FS, Yaghmai V, Berlin JW. Helical CT in the evaluation of the acute abdomen. AJR Am J Roentgenol. 2000;174:901–13.

Chapter 6
Musculoskeletal Imaging

Stephen E. Ling

Introduction

This chapter covers imaging of diseases that constitute the majority of musculoskeletal pathology: trauma, infection, neoplasm, metabolic bone disease, and arthritis. Uncommon musculoskeletal pathology, i.e., endocrine, genetic, dysplastic, and congenital disease, also require imaging but will not be discussed in this chapter. Despite a multitude of technologies available to image the musculoskeletal system, the starting point for bone pathology is typically conventional radiography (CR). Evaluation of soft tissue pathology is generally much better served by more advanced techniques, particularly magnetic resonance imaging (MRI), ultrasound (US), and at times computed tomography (CT), although occasionally CR provides significant value as well. Nuclear medicine studies are also useful in the evaluation of some musculoskeletal diseases. As with imaging any organ system, the choice of the appropriate study will depend on the clinical question to be addressed, the availability of the imaging modality, contraindications both absolute and relative, and the accuracy of the modality in balance with its risks and financial cost. With this in mind, we approach issues of imaging along lines of clinically suspected pathology. We start by reviewing the imaging armamentarium as it applies to the musculoskeletal system, including strengths and limitations, indications, and alternatives modalities.

S.E. Ling, M.D. (✉)
Department of Radiology, Temple University Hospital,
3401 N. Broad Street, Philadelphia, PA 19140, USA
e-mail: Stephen.Ling@tuhs.temple.edu

W.R. Reinus (ed.), *Clinician's Guide to Diagnostic Imaging*,
DOI 10.1007/978-1-4614-8769-2_6, © Springer Science+Business Media New York 2014

Imaging Modalities: Overview

Conventional Radiography/Plain Radiography

Although sometimes viewed as outdated and of little utility, radiographs serve as the starting point in the imaging diagnosis of many categories of suspected musculoskeletal pathology, especially trauma, osteomyelitis, focal mass lesions, and arthropathies. Plain radiographs are inexpensive, widely available, and rapidly and readily obtainable, even by the bedside if necessary.

Ultrasound

US can be used to visualize tendon pathology to good advantage, e.g., pathology of rotator cuff tendons and ankle tendons. US also is becoming a valuable tool in early inflammatory arthritis, particularly in cases of undifferentiated, unclassified inflammatory arthritis. Ultrasound can demonstrate inflammatory changes in the soft tissues, e.g., synovitis, tenosynovitis, enthesitis, and show evidence of joint destruction, i.e., erosions. In addition, application of Doppler US permits visualization of a lesion's vascularity.

US permits real time imaging, which allows for provocative maneuvers to detect pathology that is not well shown on static imaging studies. Examples of such provocative maneuvers using dynamic real time US include elbow flexion to elicit ulnar nerve subluxation at the cubital tunnel, hip flexion to show snapping of the iliopsoas tendon in the groin or the iliotibial band at the greater trochanter, and eccentric muscle contraction in the diagnosis of myofascial herniation.

US can also be used to guide interventional procedures for infection, arthritis, or soft tissue trauma (especially athletic overuse syndromes). Specifically, US can facilitate joint aspiration, drainage of fluid collections, and tissue biopsy, as well as injection of tendon sheaths, joints, bursae, and peritendinous soft tissues, e.g., the common extensor tendon origin at the lateral epicondyle of the elbow (tennis elbow), the gluteal tendons in the hip, and the plantar fascia at the foot.

US is operator-dependent, and nowhere is this more important than with musculoskeletal studies. This means that specifically trained imagers are needed for this type of examination. As mentioned in Chap. 1, US transducers have a narrow field of view, and so with today's scanning methods it is possible to overlook pathology. Despite these limitations, the role of musculoskeletal US continues to expand, especially the use of ultrasound guided procedures.

Computed Tomography

With the introduction of MRI, CT's role in musculoskeletal imaging has declined, particularly for soft tissue imaging. Nonetheless, CT has certain positive characteristics that make it a commonly used tool for some musculoskeletal pathology.

CT is most commonly used to evaluate bone trauma, particularly for acute fractures of the spine and pelvis, to plan operative reduction of complex fractures and fracture-dislocations, and to diagnose osseous nonunion of fractures. After intravenous contrast administration, CT also may be employed for diagnosis of soft tissue abscess. It should be noted, however, that MRI is generally better for abscess diagnosis, and so CT should be used only when MRI is unavailable or contraindicated. CT is highly sensitive for the presence of calcium and so can be used to detect and characterize matrix mineralization in osseous and soft tissue space occupying lesions.

Magnetic Resonance Imaging

MRI is a commonly performed musculoskeletal examination because it depicts soft tissue structures that cannot be resolved by other modalities. Specifically, these include ligaments, muscles, tendons, fibrocartilage, and fascia. MRI is thus the preferred modality to evaluate suspected internal derangement of joints, and certain types of extra-articular soft tissue pathology including traumatic muscle strains and contusions, soft tissue tumors and tumor-like entities, and soft tissue infectious processes most commonly abscess.

MRI has no imaging peer with respect to its ability to evaluate bone marrow. This permits diagnosis and characterization of pathology ranging from traumatic bone contusion and occult osseous fracture to marrow proliferative and marrow replacement diseases, both diffuse and focal. MRI also has the ability to demonstrate very early cortical abnormalities in cases of acute osteomyelitis, often earlier than other imaging modalities. While nuclear medicine bone scintigraphy performs almost as well, MRI has a slight edge, is more specific, and shows accompanying soft tissue abnormalities. Furthermore, MRI can visualize all of the features involved in soft tissue inflammation and joint damage in patients with inflammatory arthropathies, including active pathology early in the disease course that allows for administration of disease-modifying agents that may slow down progression and even reverse pathology.

Nuclear Medicine

Bone scintigraphy (BS), labeled WBC study, and PET and PET/CT are used most commonly in the evaluation of musculoskeletal pathology. These studies all routinely use very large fields of view that permit whole body evaluation for multifocal disease. As with numerous other nuclear medicine (NM) exams, a major advantage of BS, labeled WBC study, PET, and PET/CT is high sensitivity and high negative predictive value. On the other hand, these studies have low specificity, somewhat long exam length (especially with labeled WBC studies), and relatively limited ability to anatomically localize pathology. However, both specificity and anatomic localization of abnormalities have improved for both BS and PET with the addition of co-registered CT. Single photon emission CT (SPECT) has aided in localizing lesions on BS. NM studies employed for musculoskeletal applications are generally less expensive than MRI, with PET and PET/CT being exceptions.

Trauma

Osseous Trauma

In most cases, the imaging evaluation of acute or subacute musculoskeletal trauma commences with plain radiographs. Although CR provides little useful information about the soft tissues, it is sufficient to diagnose most fractures. In addition, radiographs obtained in different positions can be used to exclude instability, e.g., flexion and extension views of the spine to exclude ligamentous abnormalities [1].

At times, clinical suspicion of a fracture may persist despite negative radiographs. In this case, there are several options depending upon the body part in question and the age of the patient. For example, in the case of adult elbow trauma, it is usually reasonable to treat a patient suspected of having a radial head fracture but with negative radiographs conservatively using presumptive immobilization and have the patient return for repeat radiographs a week to 14 days later [2]. At this time the bone resorption related to early healing would make the previously occult fracture more apparent [3].

A conservative strategy is inadvisable for some occult fractures, particularly in weight-bearing bones. Instead, depending upon the patient's age and the time delay between the traumatic event and their presentation, other modalities, though more costly, may speed diagnosis and allow earlier definitive treatment. Two imaging studies fall into this category, radionuclide BS and MRI. While it may be tempting to do a CT scan when plain radiographs are negative, CT has relatively poor performance for diagnosis of radiographically occult acute fractures compared with BS and MRI.

BS is less expensive than MRI, but the time delay between the traumatic event and patient presentation will affect its diagnostic accuracy. In younger patients, where the vascular supply to bone is unimpeded by atherosclerosis, BS will show at least 95 % of fractures at approximately 24 h after the trauma. In older patients 48–72 h may be required to achieve this type of sensitivity [4]. So, if not enough time has passed between the traumatic episode and evaluation, it is advisable to wait before obtaining the scan or to use MRI for diagnosis.

MRI has an excellent track record with respect to diagnosing occult fractures. Nearly all compression-type fractures are visible within a few hours on MRI. It should be pointed out, however, that avulsion-type fractures may be problematic because identification of osseous trauma on MR relies heavily on visualizing marrow space edema, much more so than trabecular discontinuity. Avulsion fractures are typically small and so commonly generate little edema and hemorrhage in the marrow space of either the parent bone or the avulsed fragment [5]. Furthermore, since the avulsed fragment is often small and primarily cortical in nature, it may be difficult to identify on MRI. For example, MRI has relatively poor accuracy for diagnosis of Segond fractures of the lateral tibial rim at the knee. It is important that the requesting physician provide a detailed clinical history so that small avulsion fractures are not overlooked when an MRI has been chosen to evaluate the patient.

Although MRI is excellent for diagnosing acute occult fractures, it is by a large margin the most expensive modality in the diagnostic armamentarium. While some institutions have adopted a limited sequence, less expensive MR examination protocol to assess for fractures, this practice has not become widely used, at least in part because of constraints in billing and insurance reimbursements in today's medical practice environment.

In cases where initial radiographs are negative but there remains high clinical suspicion for occult fracture, both MRI and to a slightly lesser degree BS have a high degree of sensitivity for this diagnosis. The specificity of MRI is significantly greater given its ability to display other types of bone (e.g., osteoarthritis, bone contusion) [2] and adjacent soft tissue (e.g., muscle strain, muscle contusion, hematoma) pathology. American College of Radiology (ACR) appropriateness criteria very strongly favor MR over BS. For scaphoid and distal radius fractures, CT is recommended over BS when MRI is unavailable or contraindicated and the clinician is unable to or does not desire to immobilize the wrist and obtain 7–14 day follow-up radiographs [2] (Table 6.1).

Another problem with both BS and MRI is that many institutions, for economic reasons, do not offer these modalities 24 h a day or even every day of the week. If neither BS nor MRI is available, CT is the next best examination.

In contrast to extremity fractures, CT is used routinely in the initial evaluation of acute spine trauma. According to the National Emergency X-Radiography Utilization Study (NEXUS) criteria or Canadian C-Spine Rule (CCR) for cervical spine injury (CSI) criteria, MDCT with sagittal and coronal reconstructions is generally the preferred first imaging study for patients at high risk for fracture [1, 6]. This migration from CR to CT has occurred in part because CR only has 70 % sensitivity for cervical spine fractures. In pediatric patients less than 14 years of age where the incidence of spinal injury is lower, CR remains the initial imaging procedure of choice for acute spinal injury, in the cervical, thoracic, and lumbar spine in order to minimize radiation exposure [1, 6].

Generally, in cases where MDCT is used for initial assessment of acute spinal trauma, the entire spine should be imaged because severe trauma patients have a high incidence of multiple, noncontiguous injuries [1, 6]. It should be noted that thoracic and lumbar CT reconstructions derived from thoracic-abdomen-pelvic examinations are adequate substitutes for primary spine imaging, obviating the need for additional, formal spine CT imaging and thus avoiding unnecessary radiation dose to the patient.

Spine MRI is excellent for evaluation of patients in which there is clinical suspicion for spinal cord injury, cord compression, or ligamentous instability. Thus, MDCT of the cervical spine should be supplemented with an MRI in patients with posttraumatic myelopathy, with clinical or imaging findings worrisome for ligamentous injury,

Table 6.1 Fractures: efficacy of imaging modalities

Imaging modality	Sensitivity	Limitations
CR		Radiation exposure
		May take 7–10 days after injury to diagnose fracture
		2-D representation of 3-D information
		Sensitivity varies widely depending on anatomic location of injury
		Assumes technically well done studies that use proper MAs, kVp, etc., and include all pertinent views
CT		Radiation exposure
		Limited effectiveness in diagnosis of incomplete and non-displaced, complete fractures
MRI	95 %	Specificity less for small avulsion-type fractures that are often better detected with CR or CT
BS	95 %	Imaging not performed until 3–4 h after injection
		Usually takes 2–3 days after injury to diagnose fracture with high sensitivity in elderly adults
		Specificity less for non-acute fractures

or with a mechanically unstable spine for presurgical planning [1, 6]. In cases with clinical or imaging findings suggestive of arterial injury, MDCT of the cervical spine should typically be accompanied by CTA or MRA of the head and neck [1, 6].

In both pediatric and adult populations, the major role of CT in evaluation of extremity fractures is for surgical planning. CT provides extensive information on the 3D anatomy and spatial relationships of fracture fragments. It is able to assess whether or not a fracture involves a joint and show how much diastasis and step off is present at the articular surface [2, 3, 7, 8]. CT may occasionally provide information about tendon entrapment. Typically, it is at the orthopedist's discretion to request a planning CT once the decision has been made to operatively reduce the fracture. CT angiography can be useful to confirm arterial injury in cases where vascular compromise is clinically suspected from signs and symptoms such as abnormal pedal pulses, skin pallor, parathesias, and coolness of the extremity [9].

MRI can occasionally be of use in preoperative planning of extremity fracture reduction. Its role relates to identifying accompanying soft tissue injury [9], typically after fracture-dislocations caused by high-energy trauma, e.g., dislocation of the femorotibial joint of the knee. Here, MRI not only displays the status of the ligaments, but also of the menisci, tendon insertions, and focal articular cartilage defects.

Stress fractures frequently are difficult to visualize using CR, particularly insufficiency type stress fractures because of the associated osteopenia. The sensitivity of CR for early stress fracture detection may be as low as 15 % on initial imaging, with follow-up X-rays sensitivity increasing to only 50 % [10, 11]. Nonetheless, it is reasonable to begin the patient's evaluation with CR primarily to exclude other pathology. Often, however, an alternative study, either BS or MRI, will be required to diagnose the fracture. Both have a high degree of accuracy for this diagnosis, but MRI is generally the preferred examination because it depicts all of the anatomy and it uses no ionizing radiation. Of course, MRI is more expensive than BS, and this difference should be taken into consideration.

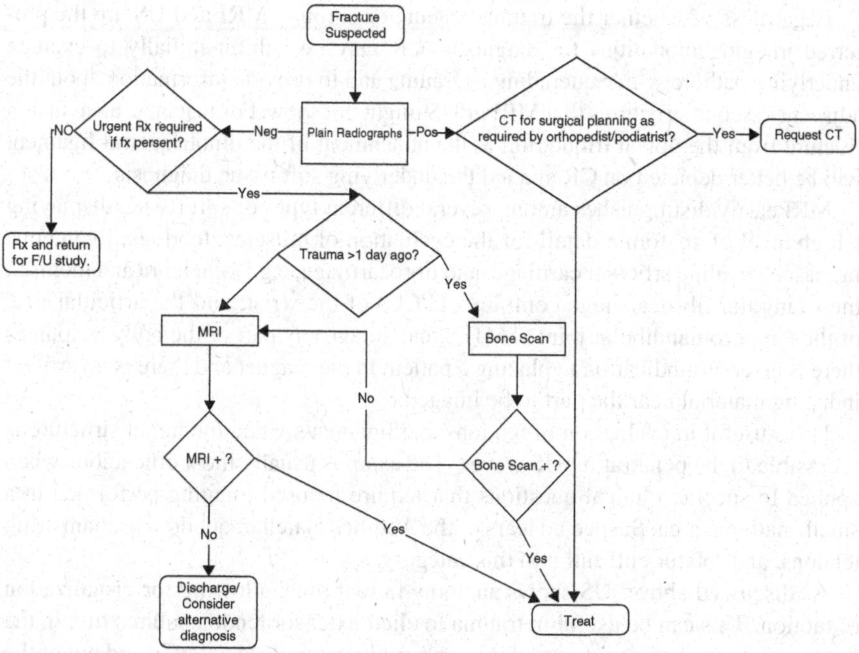

Fig. 6.1 Workup of osseous trauma

Because BS only shows abnormal metabolic activity, findings are nonspecific and always should be compared with recent CR [11, 12]. This practice will prevent incorrectly interpreting a BS abnormality as a presumed clinical diagnosis. For example, an osteoid osteoma and a stress fracture will have similar BS appearances, but these are very different entities, requiring different therapy.

US plays a limited role in initial fracture diagnosis. US, using CR as a standard, has a sensitivity and specificity of 94 % for lipohemarthrosis and hence detection of occult fractures with intra-articular extension (Fig. 6.1).

Soft Tissue Trauma

Trauma to muscles, ligaments, and tendons may occur acutely as with a sudden muscle strain or from chronic repetitive trauma, as with overuse syndromes like "tennis elbow." Other common soft tissue injuries include muscle contusions and intramuscular hematomas, cruciate ligament injury and meniscal tears in the knee, rotator cuff tears of the shoulder, shoulder glenoid and hip acetabular labral tears, carpal intrinsic ligament tears, sprains of the ankle, ankle and wrist tenosynovitis, and plantar fasciitis in the foot. Tendons, e.g., the rotator cuff, biceps at the shoulder and elbow, gluteal, hamstring, adductor, quadriceps, and Achilles tendons, may tear as a result of either acute and/or chronic trauma or as a result of other infiltrating pathology that causes degradation of the tendon's integrity, e.g., fluquinolones, xanthomas, or tophi.

Regardless of whether the trauma is acute or chronic, MRI and US are the preferred imaging modalities for diagnosis. CR may be helpful initially to exclude underlying pathology masquerading as trauma and to provide information about the adjacent osseous structures that MRI or US might not show. For instance, an avulsion fracture from the dorsal triquetrum at the attachment of the ulnotriquetral ligament will be better depicted on CR and aid the underlying soft tissue diagnosis.

MRI easily distinguishes among several different types of soft tissue, displaying a high level of anatomic detail for the evaluation of muscles, tendons, ligaments, fat, fascia, hyaline articular cartilage, and fibrocartilage, e.g., joint labra and menisci, the triangular fibrocartilage complex (TFCC) of the wrist, and the articular disc of the temporomandibular joint (TMJ). It can image any part of the body as long as there is no contraindication to placing a patient in the magnet and there is no artifact inducing material near the part to be imaged.

US is useful in evaluation of tendons and ligaments when the target structure is accessible to the penetrating US waves. The exam is usually most efficacious when applied to specific clinical questions that require focused imaging performed in a small anatomic area. Suspected tears of the Achilles, patellar, quadriceps, hamstring tendons, and rotator cuff fall into this category.

As discussed above, US shows anatomy in real time, allowing for visualization of motion. This can be useful in trauma to elicit extensor tendon subluxation in the fingers related to ligament tears, ulnar nerve subluxation-dislocation in and out of the cubital tunnel at the elbow, ankle tendon dislocations at the hind foot, and myofascial tears of muscles.

CT, in some cases, can diagnose trauma to tendons, muscles, and ligaments, but compared with MRI, its capability is limited. CT suffers from poor contrast resolution in evaluating the musculoskeletal system.

Although soft tissue abnormalities, both traumatic and non-traumatic, occasionally can be detected on BS, this study is not accurate enough to warrant its use for this purpose. In fact, these findings typically are noted incidentally on a BS obtained for a different purpose (Fig. 6.2).

Infection

Osseous Infection (Osteomyelitis)

Osteomyelitis is common in certain populations, e.g., diabetics. The vast majority (>90 %) of pediatric cases of osteomyelitis arise through hematogenous dissemination of the infectious agent, usually *Staphylococcus aureus* [13, 14]. Adult osteomyelitis, on the other hand, overwhelmingly (>90 %) results from contiguous spread of adjacent soft tissue infection, whether from a soft tissue ulcer or less commonly pyomyositis [13]. A small proportion of osteomyelitis in adults results from hematogenous spread [13]. This occurs most commonly in patients who have large intravascular boli of organisms, e.g., intravenous drug users (IVDA) in whom the spine

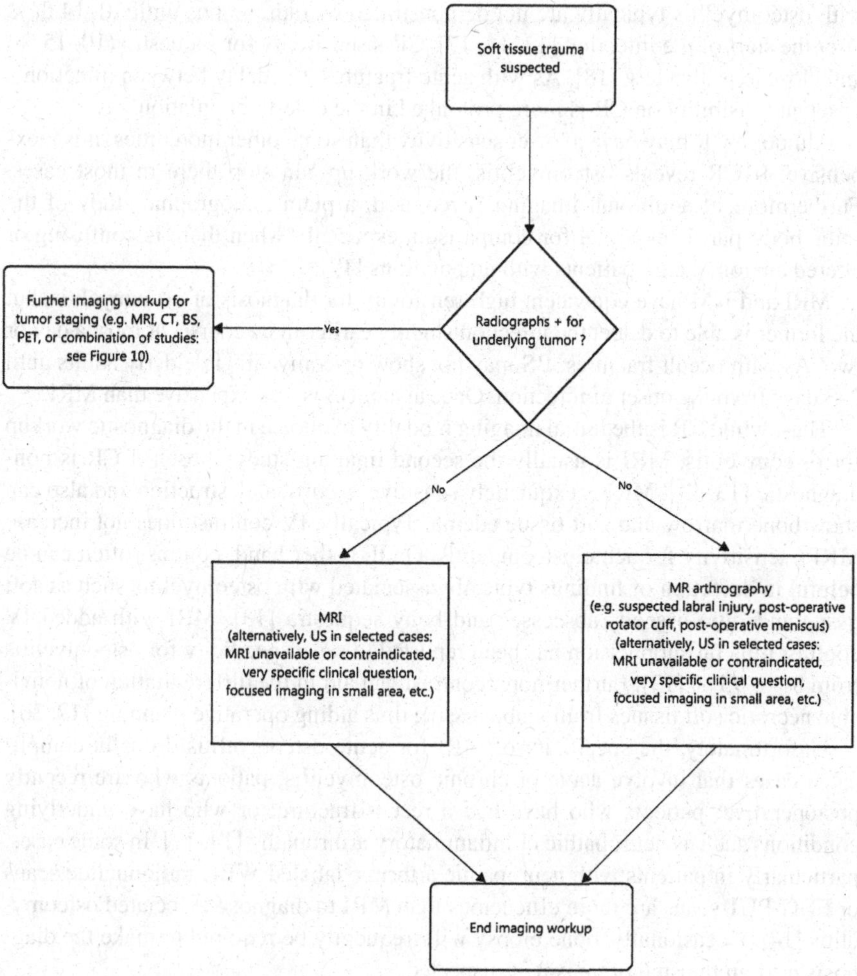

Fig. 6.2 Workup of soft tissue trauma

and sternoclavicular and acromioclavicular joints are common sites of infection [13, 15]. Osteomyelitis in any bone can spread to adjacent joints and cause septic arthritis [13, 16].

Of course, imaging can be employed not only to diagnose osteomyelitis, but also to evaluate healing in response to treatment. Finally, CR is valuable in defining postoperative anatomy in patients who have had normal anatomy altered either surgically or from neuropathic arthropathy.

Although the specificity of CR for osteomyelitis is moderately high (80 %), its sensitivity is low (54 %). The low sensitivity results from the fact that there must be substantial trabecular bone destruction for osteomyelitis to be evident on plain radiographs, usually 50–70 % [14]. As a result, the destructive changes associated with osteomyelitis typically are not demonstrated by radiographs until 10–14 days after the start of the infection [13, 14, 17]. CR's sensitivity for sequestra (10–15 %) and cloacae is also low [18]. As with acute fractures, the delay between infection's onset and visibility on CR is more prolonged in the elderly population.

Although CR may have a lower sensitivity than some other modalities, it is inexpensive. If CR reveals osteomyelitis, the work up can stop there in most cases. Furthermore, if additional imaging is required, a plain radiographic study of the same body part is essential for comparison, especially when there is confusing or altered anatomy, e.g., patients with amputations [17].

MRI and NM have equivalent high sensitivity for diagnosis of osteomyelitis, but the former is able to detect the infection slightly earlier in its course, at most a day or two. As with occult fractures, BS may not show osteomyelitis in elderly adults until 2–3 days from the onset of infection. Once again, BS is less expensive than MRI.

Thus, while CR is the initial imaging modality of choice in the diagnostic workup for osteomyelitis, MRI is usually the second imaging study chosen if CR is nondiagnostic [13, 14]. MRI is exquisitely sensitive to cortical destruction and also can show bone marrow and soft tissue edema. Typically, IV contrast does not increase MRI's sensitivity for acute osteomyelitis. On the other hand, contrast often can be helpful in detection of findings typically associated with osteomyelitis such as soft tissue and intra-osseous abscesses and bony sequestra [13]. MRI with added IV contrast plus fat suppression has been reported to raise specificity for osteomyelitis from 81 to 93 % [19]. Furthermore, contrast can aid in the differentiation of nonviable necrotic soft tissues from viable tissue, thus aiding operative planning [17, 20].

Unfortunately, the specificity of MRI for acute osteomyelitis drops in complicated cases that involve acute or chronic osteomyelitis; patients who are recently postoperative; patients who have had a recent fracture; or who have underlying conditions such as neuropathic or inflammatory arthropathy [14, 17]. In some cases, particularly in patients with neuropathic arthritis, labeled WBC radionuclide scans or FDG-PET scans are more efficacious than MRI to diagnose associated osteomyelitis [14]. Occasionally, bone biopsy will frequently be required to make the diagnosis or if an unusual organism is suspected.

Findings on follow-up MRI studies in patients with osteomyelitis routinely lag the clinical picture, and so can give an incorrect impression of the status of patients who are undergoing or recently had treatment. Findings on MRI such as marrow edema and marrow enhancement may worsen during the treatment phase, not showing improvement until later on. Regardless, evidence of progressive bone destruction should not be evident and indicates worsening infection.

In patients who are unable to have MRI, whether due to unavailability of or contraindication to the exam, BS may be used instead. As mentioned, BS has equally high sensitivity for detection of osteomyelitis as MRI and as a result has extremely high negative predictive value; a negative study virtually excludes osteomyelitis [14]. In addition, BS allows imaging of the entire skeleton, making it valuable in cases of suspected multifocal infection such as chronic recurrent multifocal osteomyelitis. The main drawbacks of BS are its inability to detect infection as early as MRI, and its lower specificity compared with MRI, CR, and other studies [14]. The development of single photon emission CT (SPECT) in registration with standard CT has mitigated some of these issues but also has increased the cost of nuclear medicine studies substantially. In some special circumstances, such as cases of multifocal osteomyelitis and osteomyelitis around prostheses, BS combined with labeled WBC study can be particularly beneficial; the labeled WBC study improves the low specificity of BS alone [17]. Labeled WBC studies are most useful in the appendicular skeleton. Many studies have shown problems with false negatives and low sensitivity for osteomyelitis of the spine evaluated with labeled WBC [21].

Diagnosing ongoing chronic osteomyelitis can be difficult. Early studies using FDG-PET showed higher sensitivity and specificity than other NM studies and MRI both [14]. A recent meta-analysis that reviewed the accuracy of multiple imaging modalities for the diagnosis of chronic osteomyelitis showed FDG-PET to be the most accurate, with a sensitivity of 96 % and specificity of 91 %. In comparison, the sensitivity and specificity of MRI was 84 % and 60 %, respectively. Labeled WBC study had a sensitivity of 84 % and a specificity of 80 %, but these values decreased considerably when cases involving the axial skeleton were included [22]. Relative unavailability and high cost are significant stumbling blocks for FDG-PET.

Although MRI often can diagnose a sequestrum, CT is slightly more sensitive because it is exquisitely sensitive for detecting calcification and ossification [13]. CT is especially applicable if the suspected sequestrum is small or IV contrast cannot be administered with the MRI [13, 14]. On the other hand, if a patient can tolerate IV contrast, MRI is superior to CT in determination of the viability of infected bone, and even more accurate than CT in the detection of necrotic soft tissues that may require surgical debridement [13, 17].

In selected locations in the body where radiographs do not display the anatomy clearly CT is the preferred initial examination in cases of suspected osteomyelitis, e.g., sternoclavicular joints [13, 14]. CT also may be preferred in areas where respiratory motion may degrade MRI image quality, e.g., the chest and abdominal walls [23, 24]. CT, if positive, is capable of providing precise anatomic localization of osteomyelitis. It also is able to guide bone biopsy. CT is very limited in evaluation of the marrow space compared with MRI [14, 17] (Table 6.2).

US plays a minor role in the diagnosis of osteomyelitis. The modality cannot detect intra-osseous pathology such as medullary bone destruction, sequestrum, and intra-osseous abscess [14, 17]. US does have very good utility in the detection of infection of the soft tissues adjacent to infected bone and periosteal abnormalities primarily in children. For instance, US can identify periosteal elevation and accompanying subperiosteal fluid collections such as abscess, and it also is able to demonstrate neighboring soft tissue abscesses in patients with osteomyelitis [14]. In addition, in cases where osteomyelitis is intra-capsular in location, such as the femoral neck, US has high sensitivity in detection of joint effusion, but it cannot distinguish whether the effusion reflects complicating septic arthritis or is merely reactive in etiology [14]. US, like CT, can provide guidance for aspiration of fluid collections and joint effusions related to osteomyelitis (Fig. 6.3).

Table 6.2 Osteomyelitis: efficacy of imaging modalities

Imaging modality	Sensitivity	Specificity	Accuracy	Advantages	Limitations
CR	54 % (22–93 %)	80 % (50–94 %)		May demonstrate an alternative diagnosis (i.e., fracture nonunion, tumor)	Radiation exposure
				Excellent overview and delineation of anatomy (especially beneficial in postoperative and neuroarthropathy patients)	2-D representation of 3-D information
				Aids characterization of the distribution of arthritic changes (including neuropathic osteoarthropathy)	Usually takes 10–14 days after infection onset to diagnose osteomyelitis
				Useful in detection of soft tissue gas	Bone destruction needed for visualization of the abnormality may be 60 %
				Specificity moderate	Sensitivity low to very low
				—	
					Endplate cortical destruction in osteomyelitis-discitis usually not evident until at least 4–6 weeks after infection onset
					Specificity in spondylodiscitis reduced by other causes of disc space narrowing (e.g., DDD), endplate erosive changes (e.g., severe DDD), and gross bone destruction (e.g., neuropathic spondyloarthropathy, amyloid arthropathy)

CT		Helpful in evaluation of deep structures and assessment of atypical and irregular bones and joints, and complex joint anatomy (e.g., sternum, sternoclavicular joint, spine, pelvis)	Radiation exposure
		Precise anatomic localization of findings	Soft tissue contrast moderate, but lower than MRI
		Depicts subtle, early bone cortex erosion	Much less sensitivity for marrow infection (vs. MRI)
		Very good for sequestrum detection	
		Can guide bone biopsy	Insensitive, inadequate assessment of degree of marrow involvement
			Accuracy in determination of viability of infected bone and soft tissues lower than MRI
			—
			Inferior soft tissue contrast resolution results in decreased sensitivity for epidural abscess complicating spondylodiscitis

(continued)

Table 6.2 (continued)

Imaging modality	Sensitivity	Specificity	Accuracy	Advantages	Limitations
MRI	92 % (29–100 %)	84 % (78–89 %)	89–98%[a]	Comprehensive assessment of entire spectrum of bone and soft tissue infection pathology	Not always (easily) available
	84%[a]	60%[a]		Excellent bone marrow evaluation	Expensive
				Outstanding soft tissue contrast aids diagnosis of coexisting pathology (e.g., soft tissue abscess, sinus tract, devitalized soft tissue)	Long study length may result in image quality degraded by motion artifact (difficult for severely ill patients to remain in scanner entire study)
				Superb anatomic detail	Nephrogenic systemic fibrosis (NSF) risk from IV gadolinium-based contrast agents (GBCAs)
				Provides surgeon with preoperative anatomic "road map" of pathology	Specificity decreased in setting of recent fracture, recent surgery, neuropathic osteoarthropathy, and inflammatory arthritis
				Sensitivity and specificity high (>90 %)	Nonspecific result is not uncommon but may help in evaluation of complex cases of chronic osteomyelitis
				May help in evaluation of complex cases of chronic osteomyelitis but nonspecific result is not uncommon	—
				—	Limited ability to accurately differentiate pyogenic vs. mycobacterial etiology in osteomyelitis-discitis
				Highest sensitivity (96 %), specificity (92 %), and accuracy (94 %) modality for spondylodiscitis	
BS	91 % (69–95 %)	46 % (38–100 %)		Allows for evaluation of entire body (particularly helpful with multifocal osteomyelitis)	Usually takes 2–3 days after infection onset to diagnose osteomyelitis in elderly adults
				Sensitivity high (equal to MRI)	Moderate study length (images obtained 3–4 h after radiotracer injection)
				Negative predictive value (NPV) high	Specificity very low
					Low resolution, suboptimal anatomic localization (but improved by SPECT or CT)

Labeled WBC	86 % (45–100 %)	84 % (67–89 %)	78–90 %	Allows for evaluation of entire body (particularly helpful with multifocal osteomyelitis)	Very long study length (imaging performed 2–4, 24, and possibly 48 h after injection)
	84%[a]	80%[a]		Sensitivity high	Specificity reduced in setting of recent fracture, recent surgery, neuropathic osteoarthropathy, and inflammatory arthritis
				Negative predictive value (NPV) high	Sensitivity for vertebral osteomyelitis much lower than for bone infection in the extremities
				—	
				NM commonly favored in setting of postoperative spondylodiscitis because of reduced specificity of MRI	Low resolution, suboptimal anatomic localization (but improved by SPECT or CT)
BS+labeled WBC	88 % (73–100 %)	82 % (55–91 %)	81 %	Allows for evaluation of entire body (particularly helpful with multifocal osteomyelitis)	Very long study length (imaging performed 2–4, 24, and possibly 48 h after injection)
				Sensitivity high	Specificity reduced in setting of recent fracture, recent surgery, neuropathic osteoarthropathy, and inflammatory arthritis
				Negative predictive value (NPV) high	Low resolution, suboptimal anatomic localization (but improved by SPECT or CT)
				Specificity of BS increased by addition of labeled WBC study, and vice versa	
				—	
				NM commonly favored in setting of postoperative spondylodiscitis because of reduced specificity of MRI	
FDG-PET	96%[a]	91%[a]	94 %[a]	Allows for evaluation of entire body (particularly helpful with multifocal osteomyelitis)	Relative lack of availability
				Sensitivity and specificity high	High cost
				Negative predictive value (NPV) high	—
				Particularly useful in difficult, complex cases of chronic osteomyelitis (vs. any modality)	Not reliable for osteomyelitis-discitis even though addition of CT increases specificity
				—	
				NM commonly favored in postoperative spondylodiscitis setting because of reduced specificity of MRI	
Probe to bone	66 %	85 %			Presence of granulation tissue over ulcer very uncommon but may give false negative result

[a]Chronic osteomyelitis

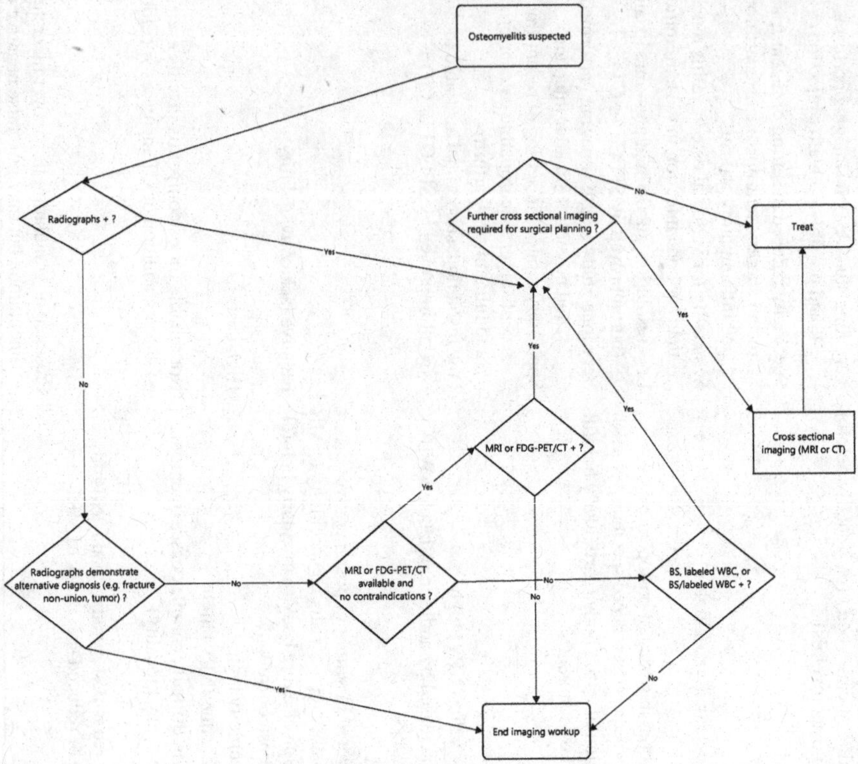

Fig. 6.3 Workup of osseous infection (osteomyelitis)

Spinal Infection (Osteomyelitis-Discitis, Spondylodiscitis)

Spinal osteomyelitis and discitis represents only approximately 5 % of all cases of osteomyelitis. Spondylodiscitis occurs most frequently in the lumbosacral spine. Cervical spine involvement is least common. Epidural spread is not uncommon but is a source of significant morbidity and mortality. Rarely, the infection spreads to the meninges and spinal cord, usually with devastating results [25]. As in the case of patients with extra-spinal osteomyelitis, bacterial infection is much more common than fungal or parasitic etiologies, and again *S. aureus* is the most common causative organism, accounting for more than half of cases (60 %) [25]. Gram negative pyogenic and polymicrobial infection is also frequently seen. *Mycobacterium* infection, including *M. tuberculosis,* is another common etiology, particularly in developing countries, where it is widespread and even endemic [25].

As with evaluation of osteomyelitis elsewhere, CR is the first study for imaging patients with suspected osteomyelitis-discitis. As with other locations, the sensitivity of X-rays for spondylitis is low, especially early in the course of the disease.

In adults, endplate cortical destruction, the most specific finding for pyogenic infection, is usually not evident on radiographs until at least 4–6 weeks after the onset of infection [25]. The sensitivity of radiographs for spinal infections for non-pyogenic osteomyelitis-discitis is worse—minimal to none. CR also has limited specificity for discitis-osteomyelitis [25]. Overall, disc space narrowing is most frequently the result of degenerative disc disease and occasionally even erosion and irregularity may be seen in severe degenerative disc disease. Gross bone destruction and osseous fragmentation can be the result of amyloid spondyloarthropathy and neuropathic arthropathy [25].

MRI is the gold standard in imaging of spinal infection [13, 25]. Numerous studies have shown that MRI has very high sensitivity, specificity, and accuracy for osteomyelitis-discitis, approximately 96 %, 92 %, and 94 %, respectively. These figures exceed those of any other imaging modality [25]. MRI's performance in detection of bone and disc infection stems from its excellent depiction of disc fluid, endplate cortical erosion, overt bone destruction, and bone marrow edema. It is also sensitive for identification of associated inflammatory phlegmon and abscess, usually either epidural or retroperitoneal within the psoas muscle. These usually require drainage for successful treatment. IV contrast can provide additional value, providing better delineation of fluid collections and improved detection of necrotic tissue and sequestra.

CT is sometimes beneficial in the workup of osteomyelitis-discitis. Like MRI, CT is capable of providing precise anatomic localization and detail in osteomyelitis-discitis. As expected, however, CT is beset by the same disadvantages relative to MRI as in the diagnosis of osteomyelitis outside the spine. Unless MRI is unavailable or contraindicated, CT is generally no longer used for this diagnosis.

NM studies play a small role in the initial diagnosis of osteomyelitis-discitis except in postoperative patients where distinction between operative changes and infection is difficult on MRI [25]. As with extra-axial infection, BS and labeled WBC studies either alone or in combination are typically used in postoperative patients. PET has not proven to be dependable in the diagnosis of spondylodiscitis, although the addition of CT improves anatomic localization and specificity (Fig. 6.4).

Joint Infection (Septic Arthritis)

In the clinical setting of a single acutely painful joint, septic arthritis should be strongly considered and evaluated emergently to avoid rapid irreversible destruction of the joint [26]. Septic arthritis in children typically arises from hematogenous inoculation of the joint, while in adults it arises from direct inoculation of the joint. Osteomyelitis that is intracapsular to a joint also can give rise to septic arthritis [13, 16].

Certain patient populations have a predilection to develop septic arthritis, in particular anatomic locations. For instance, in IVDA, the acromioclavicular joints,

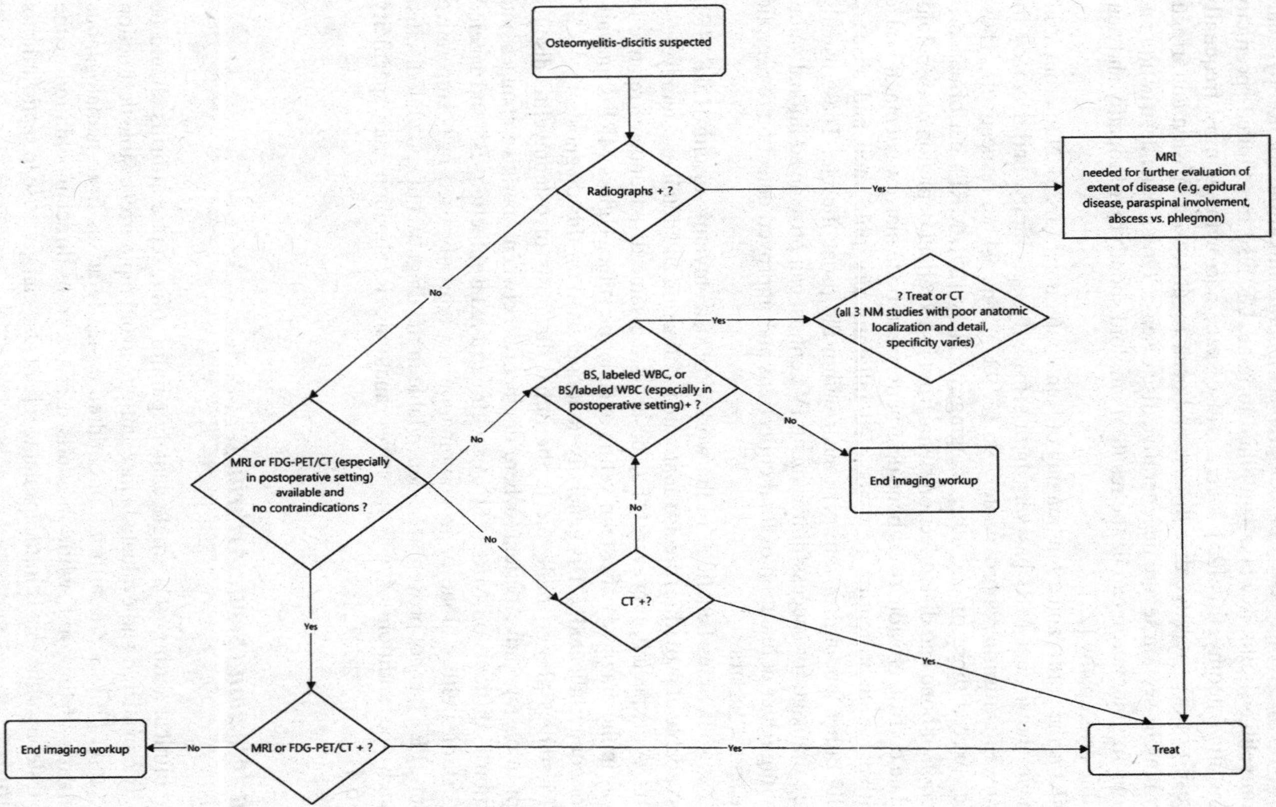

Fig. 6.4 Workup of spinal infection (osteomyelitis-discitis, spondylodiscitis)

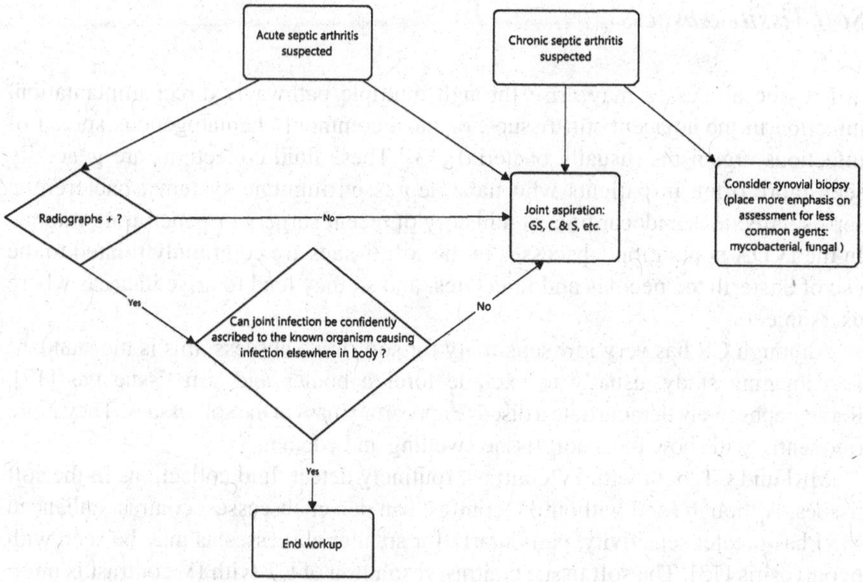

Fig. 6.5 Workup of joint infection (septic arthritis)

sternoclavicular joints, vertebral discs, and sacroiliac joints are commonly involved [15]. Patients within 6 months of arthroplasty are also prone to infection.

Joint aspiration remains the gold standard in the diagnosis of acute septic arthritis [13, 26]. MRI and US can confirm the presence of joint fluid prior to joint aspiration, but they cannot reliably distinguish sterile joint fluid from infected joint fluid [26]. In fact, routine imaging cannot exclude septic arthritis even with a normal examination [13]. Regardless, both MRI and US are only occasionally performed and almost always are unnecessary since they do not obviate the need for joint aspiration [13]. On the other hand, fluoroscopy and US can be useful to guide joint aspiration procedures. When there is clinical concern for chronic septic arthritis, in the majority of patients joint aspiration remains the initial examination. However, one should at least consider performing synovial biopsy, placing more emphasis on evaluation for less common infectious agents such as mycobacteria and fungi [26].

To summarize, although laboratory results may be normal in an acutely infected joint, clinical data, i.e., elevated CRP, sedimentation rate, leukocytosis, fever, systemic infection, and joint pain, should be emphasized over and pursued earlier than most imaging studies. Judicious use of advanced imaging techniques such as MRI, US, and nuclear medicine may help exclude alternative diagnoses, but joint aspiration and culture is the examination of choice in cases of septic arthritis (Fig. 6.5).

Soft Tissue Abscess

Soft tissue abscesses may arise through multiple pathways: direct implantation, infection in the adjacent soft tissues, or most commonly hematogenous spread of infectious organisms (usually bacteria) [13]. These fluid collections are generally seen more often in patients who have depressed immune systems, bacteremia, sepsis, infectious endocarditis, or a history of recent surgery or penetrating trauma. In the IVDA population, abscesses in the soft tissues are commonly related to the use of unsterilized needles and injectates, and so they tend to arise in areas where users inject.

Although CR has very low sensitivity for soft tissue abscess, this is the standard first imaging study, usually to exclude foreign bodies and soft tissue gas [17]. Radiographs rarely demonstrate a discrete appearing mass in the soft tissues. They more frequently will show focal soft tissue swelling and edema.

MRI and CT, both with IV contrast, routinely detect fluid collections in the soft tissues. Although MRI without IV contrast can detect abscesses, contrast enhanced MRI has greater sensitivity, particularly for smaller abscesses as may be seen with pyomyositis [13]. The soft tissue contrast resolution of CT with IV contrast is moderate and inferior to that of MRI. Moreover, depending on the timing of CT image acquisition relative to administration of the IV contrast, the fluid collection may have poor conspicuity and go undetected. Therefore, MRI with IV contrast is the preferred examination for diagnosis of a soft tissue abscess [13, 17, 26]. In addition to its utility in evaluation for soft tissue abscesses, MRI can characterize the extent of tissue devitalization and so facilitate operative planning for soft tissue debridement or amputation [17, 20].

Abscesses are also easily diagnosed with targeted US. Using color Doppler, US can add further value in some cases by assessing the vascularity of the wall of the collection and adjacent soft tissues. The presence of hypervascularity in the wall and surrounding soft tissue favors a diagnosis of abscess over a noninfected collection such as seroma or hematoma [17]. It should be cautioned, however, that there can be significant overlap in the vascularity and central echogenicity of these different types of fluid collections because seromas and hematomas can become superinfected. As a result, fluid aspiration often is needed for definitive diagnosis. Both CT and US can provide excellent guidance for this procedure [17, 27].

The differential diagnosis of soft tissue abscess on MRI, CT, and US includes muscle infarction and necrotic tumor [28]. Differentiating between abscess and necrotic tumor often can be done clinically. On the other hand, distinguishing between abscess and muscle infarction, most commonly seen as a complication of diabetes, typically requires aspiration to determine the cause of the collection.

Labeled WBC study for soft tissue abscess is less often utilized than MRI, CT and US because it provides limited anatomic localization of abscesses [29]. Furthermore, labeled WBC exams take much longer to perform than other modalities, and this can be a problem in acutely ill patients or because it can increase an inpatient's length-of-stay. Nonetheless it has high sensitivity and excellent specificity for abscess (Table 6.3, Fig. 6.6).

Table 6.3 Soft tissue abscess: efficacy of imaging modalities

Imaging modality	Sensitivity	Specificity	Limitations
CR	+	+++++	Radiation exposure Poor soft tissue evaluation Finding of discrete soft tissue fluid collection/mass only occasionally seen, with collection + internal air or air fluid level rare
US	++++/+++++	++++	Specificity mildly reduced by other possible fluid collections (e.g., hematoma, seroma)
CT (with IV contrast)	+++/++++	++++	Radiation exposure Soft tissue contrast less than MRI Peripheral, rim-like wall enhancement dependent on appropriate timing of IV contrast injection
MRI (without and with IV contrast)	++++/+++++	++++	Not always (readily) available Expensive Long study length may result in image quality degraded by motion artifact (difficult for very ill patients to remain in scanner for complete study) Nephrogenic systemic fibrosis (NSF) risk from IV gadolinium-based contrast agents (GBCAs) Sensitivity reduced if no IV contrast (particularly with small, less conspicuous fluid collections)
Labeled WBC	++++	++++	Very long study length (imaging at 24 and possibly 48 h postinjection of labeled WBC) Limited precise anatomic localization of pathology due to low contrast resolution (better with SPECT, more recent unequivocal improvement with CT)

Pyomyositis

Known also as infectious myositis, pyomyositis is rare with higher incidence in immunocompromised patients, e.g., diabetes and AIDS [15, 16]. The disorder most often afflicts the thighs and buttocks and is multifocal in approximately 50 % of cases [15]. A minority of patients develop one or more intramuscular abscesses, often small in size [13]. If pyomyositis is not complicated by soft tissue abscess, MRI, CT, and US will typically show features of nonspecific edema and distortion of soft tissue planes, analogous to what is seen on CR.

Necrotizing Fasciitis

Necrotizing fasciitis is a fulminant and rapidly spreading infection of the tissues around the deep fascia, associated with a high degree of morbidity and mortality.

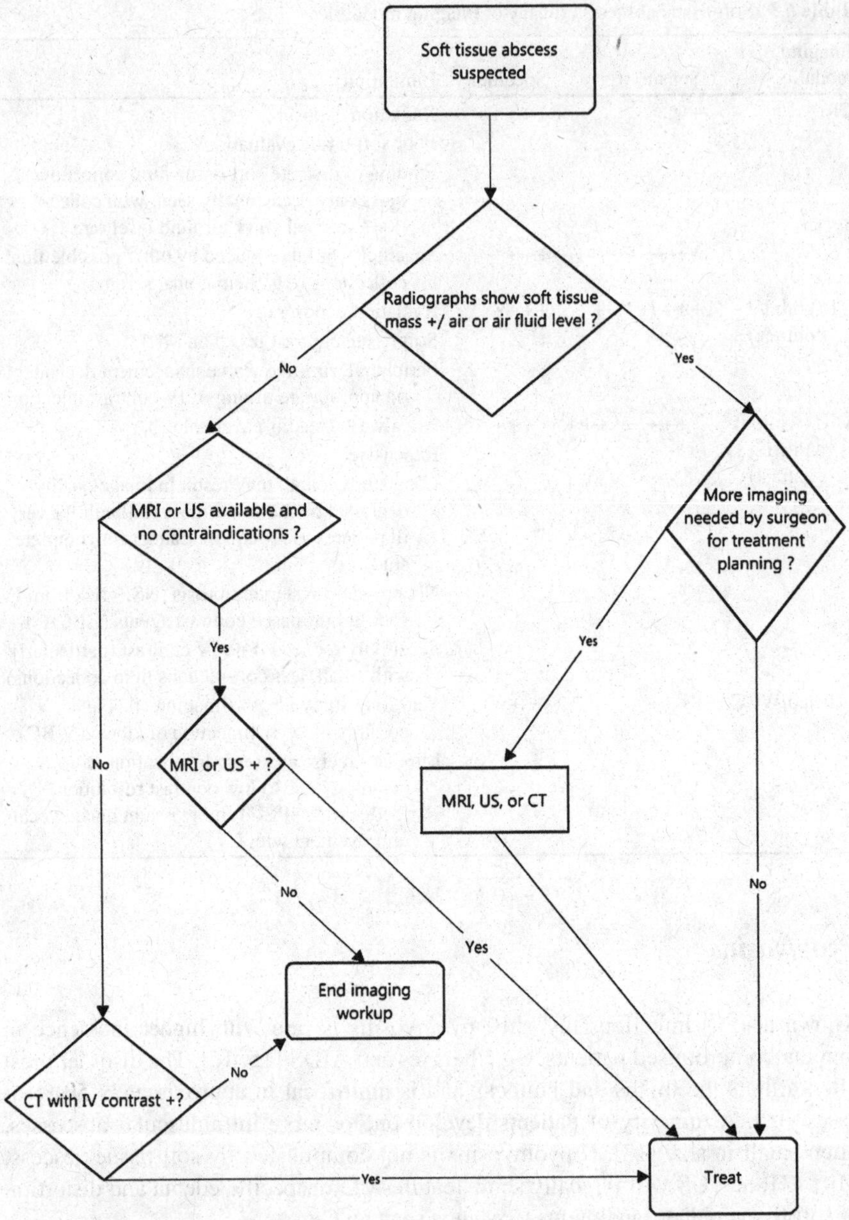

Fig. 6.6 Workup of soft tissue abscess

Given its virulent nature, prompt treatment is essential. Findings on cross-sectional imaging tend to be nonspecific until late in the disease. As a result, necrotizing fasciitis is primarily a clinical diagnosis and imaging plays a limited role in diagnosing this entity.

Neoplastic and Non-Neoplastic Space Occupying Lesions

Focal Lesions of Bone

Radiographs are indispensable in the evaluation of focal lesions of bone, whether primary neoplasms, secondary neoplasms, or non-neoplastic. In the majority of cases analysis of radiographic findings allows either a definitive diagnosis or a narrow differential diagnosis [30, 31]. In fact, radiographs are often diagnostically superior to more advanced imaging modalities, and they are invariably less expensive. Today, CR remains the gold standard for establishment of the appropriate diagnosis of tumor and tumor-like bone lesions [32]. In some cases, however, MRI and CT may provide additional information that narrows the differential diagnostic considerations. For example, a finding of multiple fluid-fluid levels in a lesion on MRI may suggest a diagnosis of aneurysmal bone cyst.

Often focal bone lesions are asymptomatic and incidentally noted on radiographs that were obtained for unrelated reasons. Many of these lesions have classic radiographic appearances and correlate with nonaggressive, benign entities that may not require additional work up, e.g., non-ossifying fibroma, mature osteochondroma, and bone island. Some lesions, although benign, may require further evaluation as they may enlarge and cause symptoms or threaten the integrity of the bone, e.g., unicameral bone cysts, aneurysmal bone cysts, giant cell tumors, and chondroblastomas. In these cases, evaluation with MRI or CT provides the anatomic detail needed for surgical planning to define the size of the lesion and what adjacent anatomic structures it impacts [32].

Sometimes a focal bone lesion is suspected clinically. If radiographs are negative, depending upon the lesion suspected, a BS, CT, or MRI may be the next imaging choice. Whether suspected or incidentally discovered on advanced imaging, CR is usually obtained to further define the nature of the lesion. If the radiographs do not adequately show the lesion or fail to make the diagnosis, CT or MRI may be required. Although most primary lesions of bone are best evaluated with MRI, CT is preferred over MRI for lesions that are juxtacortical-periosteal, located in flat bones that have thin cortices and little marrow space, and for detection and characterization of tumor matrix mineralization [32] (Fig. 6.7).

Metastases to Bone

Metastases to bone are common, occurring much more often than primary bone tumors. From 30 to 70 % of cancer patients will develop osseous metastases during the course of their illness [33]. Although many epithelial neoplasms metastasize to bone, lung, breast, prostate, renal, and thyroid malignancies are the most common.

Some malignancies, e.g., prostate cancer, have laboratory tests that can suggest progression or spread of disease, but no laboratory test is specific enough to predict

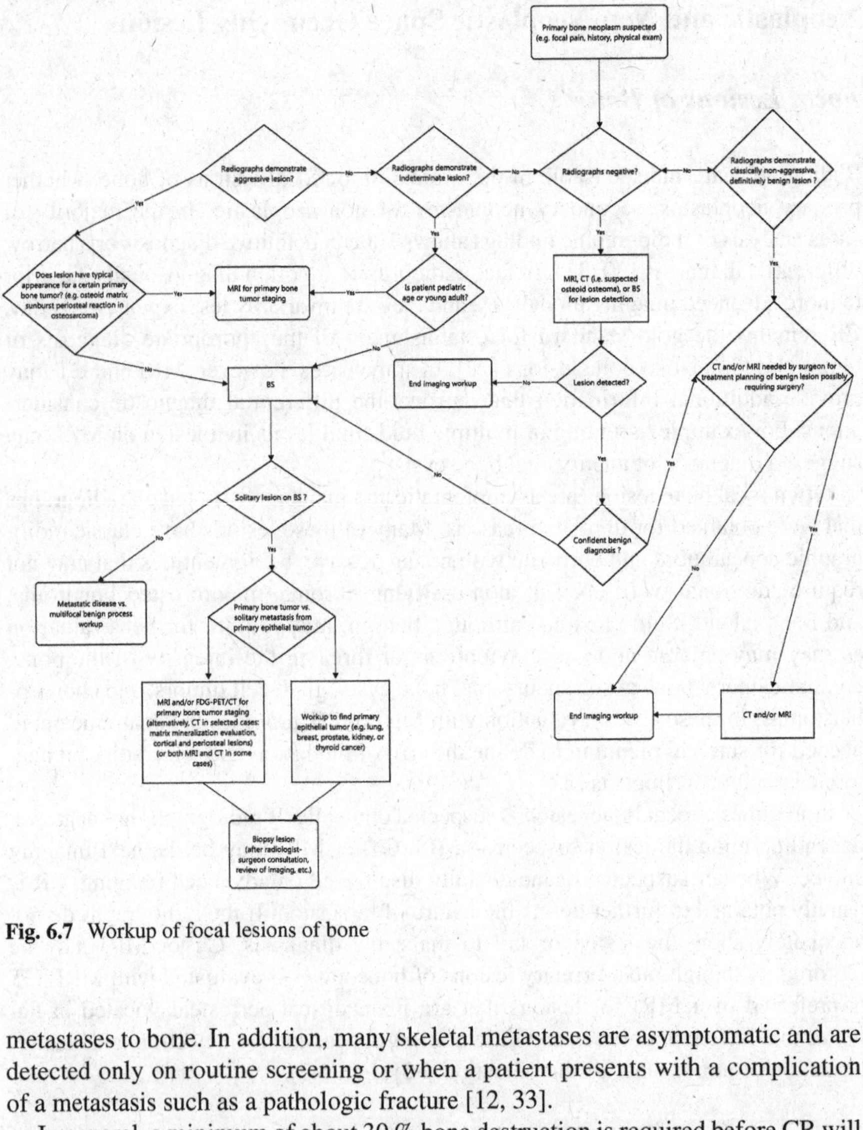

Fig. 6.7 Workup of focal lesions of bone

metastases to bone. In addition, many skeletal metastases are asymptomatic and are detected only on routine screening or when a patient presents with a complication of a metastasis such as a pathologic fracture [12, 33].

In general, a minimum of about 30 % bone destruction is required before CR will depict osteolytic lesions [34]. Some studies report even higher threshold values, 50 % [35] or even 70 % destruction. Thus, radiographs have low sensitivity for bone metastases, particularly early ones. As a result, the imaging workup for osseous metastatic disease from most epithelial malignancies begins with BS, which has been shown to have high sensitivity for this use. BS is most effective for osteoblastic metastases, the majority of which arise from breast or prostate cancer. The sensitivity of BS for osteolytic metastases is lower than for blastic metastases, particularly with renal and thyroid cancer where the lesions are often highly destructive. Nevertheless, BS's sensitivity for detection of osteolytic metastases is high (86 %) [33].

For primary malignancies that uncommonly or rarely metastasize to the skeletal system, e.g., gastrointestinal and gynecological malignancies, BS is usually obtained at time of initial presentation only when there is evidence of advanced disease [36]. Thus, BS currently forms the mainstay of initial screening for metastatic disease as well as a part of routine follow-up of cancer patients.

BS has the advantage of imaging the entire skeleton. This is important since nearly 15 % of bone metastases occur in locations in the appendicular skeleton not routinely imaged on a skeletal survey [12]. Today, newer imaging techniques such as whole body (WB) MRI, PET, and PET/CT are able to evaluate nearly the entire skeleton on a single study. On meta-analysis BS has moderate to high specificity in detection of osseous metastases on a per-patient basis with overall sensitivity and specificity of 86 % and 81 %, respectively. Even so both MRI (91 and 95 %) and FDG-PET (90 and 97 %) exhibit higher sensitivity and specificity than BS [33]. Thus far, however, BS remains the mainstay of work up because it is low cost and is nearly as sensitive as more expensive examinations.

Although some patterns of abnormality on BS clearly indicate metastases, others are nonspecific. As a result, when areas of abnormal radionuclide uptake are discovered on a BS done to exclude metastases, comparison radiographs are required to exclude benign pathology, such as degenerative disc disease, as the etiology of the BS abnormality [33]. This means that if no benign explanation or no abnormality at all is visible on CR, the BS lesion is taken to represent a metastasis, and further work up must be pursued.

A solitary lesion on BS in patients with a known primary epithelial malignancy is common. The frequency varies with the type of primary malignancy and the location of the BS abnormality. For example, such a finding in the rib cage reflects a bone metastasis approximately 25 % (range: 10–40 %) of the time [37]. More often than not, the BS finding will require additional evaluation with radiographs. If these are unrevealing, MRI, PET, and/or PET-CT may be required [12]. Similarly, this protocol can be applied to BS studies showing multiple foci of abnormal uptake. Biopsy may be necessary in some of the cases in which imaging is diagnostically inconclusive [12].

Most primary malignancies of bone, as opposed to epithelial cancers, do not metastasize to other skeletal sites and so BS is not indicated. On the other hand, both osteosarcoma and Ewing's sarcoma often do spread to other skeletal sites, and so BS is a necessary part of the evaluation in patients with these tumors [12].

The main role of CT in the evaluation of a bone metastasis is to determine whether the lesion has caused enough cortical destruction to put the bone at risk for pathologic fracture [32]. CT is insensitive at detecting malignant marrow infiltration and so has only low to moderate sensitivity for osseous metastatic involvement [33]. As a result, it is not used for screening or evaluation of most lesions.

MRI is an excellent imaging choice for assessment of the bone marrow [32, 38] and will show osseous metastases that do not involve the cortex. In fact, as mentioned above, (WB) MRI has specificity and sensitivity that is equal to or greater than that of BS and FDG-PET/CT. Even so, BS is favored by current ACR guidelines over MRI [12]. As such, MRI is a good staging tool, but has little value in screening.

MRI, because of its high sensitivity to bone infiltration, has a tendency to overestimate the amount of cortical destruction a metastasis has caused. As a result, it poorly predicts if a metastasis is of orthopedic significance. Also, conventional MRI has a poor track record when it comes to distinguishing acute traumatic or osteoporotic compression fractures from pathologic fractures in the spine. Some have suggested that MRI with diffusion-weighted imaging may be more effective at differentiating between benign and malignant vertebral collapse, but this technique is still under investigation [12].

Finally, ACR Appropriateness Criteria state that MRI for metastatic bone disease does not require administration of IV contrast. Vertebral metastases form an exception because here IV contrast can help to outline soft tissue extension. Regardless, IV contrast tends to be useful in the evaluation of primary soft tissue lesions [12, 39].

FDG-PET has high contrast resolution and allows for whole body evaluation. In addition, unlike most other imaging modalities, it provides information about metabolic activity [32]. As such, it provides both morphologic and physiologic information. FDG-PET is better at identifying osteolytic or mixed lytic and blastic metastases than those that are purely blastic. This explains why BS remains the screening test of choice for osteoblastic bone metastases [33, 40, 41] (Table 6.4, Fig. 6.8).

Multiple Myeloma

Multiple myeloma (MM), including its cousin plasmacytoma, is the most common primary malignancy of bone. Although MM commonly causes lytic lesions in bone, it has some unique features that deserve elucidation. Histomorphometric studies have shown uncoupled or severely imbalanced bone remodeling with increased bone resorption and decreased or absent bone formation in patients with multiple myeloma. Specifically there is stimulation of osteoclast formation and activity in close proximity to myeloma cells. Concurrently, myeloma cells suppress osteoblasts and thereby inhibit bone formation. In addition to blocking osteoblast formation and inhibiting osteoblast function, myeloma cells have also been reported to up-regulate osteoblast apoptosis [34]. Nearly 10 % of MM patients present with diffuse osteopenia on CR at the time of diagnosis [34]. The remaining patients are either radiographically normal or have visible lytic lesions. Eventually, as many as 90 % of MM patients will develop osteolytic lesions [34].

Only about 50 % of myeloma lesions are detected by BS, making it inappropriate as a screening tool for active MM. As a result, skeletal survey (SS), a radiographic technique that images nearly the entire skeleton, traditionally has been the test used to diagnose and follow patients with MM. As in the case of osseous metastatic disease, extensive destruction of bone, between 30 and 75 %, must be present before myeloma lesions become evident on SS [42, 43]. Despite the diagnostic limitations of SS, as recently as in 2009, the International Myeloma Working Group (IMWG) issued a consensus statement on the role of imaging techniques in multiple myeloma in which whole body X-ray, i.e., SS, was considered the standard for initial staging of MM [34, 42].

Table 6.4 Bone metastases: efficacy of imaging modalities[a]

Imaging modality	Sensitivity[a]	Specificity[a]	Limitations
CR			Sensitivity very low Especially limited in areas of overlapping structures, deep locations, and anatomically complex bones and joints
CT	73 % (77 %)	95 % (83 %)	Insensitive, inadequate assessment of marrow involvement Sensitivity moderate but comparatively low (vs. MRI, BS, FDG-PET)
MRI[b]	91 % (90 %)	95 % (96 %)	Whole body (WB) MRI specificity and sensitivity equal to or greater than each of BS and FDG-PET/CT separately, but either BS (i.e., initial presentation breast cancer) or FDG-PET/CT (i.e., initial presentation breast cancer with negative BS, or known bone metastases with pathologic femur fracture) may be favored by current ACR guidelines over MRI in some instances Limited quantification of cortical bone destruction (vs. CT)
BS[c]	86 % (75 %)	81 % (94 %)	Sensitivity reduced by false negatives resulting from rapidly growing, near purely osseous metastases (e.g., renal, thyroid) Specificity reduced by high false positive rate caused by increased turnover of bone in numerous benign primary bone tumors, non-neoplastic lesions, fractures, and degenerative disease Worse accuracy than FDG-PET/CT overall Preferred over FDG-PET for osteoblastic metastases "Flare" effect on follow-up imaging after therapy can be misleading in patients with positive response to treatment
FDG-PET[d]	90 % (87 %)	97 % (97 %)	Sensitivity for detection of osteoblastic metastases lower than for osteolytic and mixed lytic/blastic lesions FDG-PET/CT better than FDG-PET

[33] Meta-analysis—67 articles, 145 studies, 1995–2010

[a]On per-patient basis (per-lesion basis)

[b]Includes both conventional axial and whole body MRI, and both unenhanced and contrast enhanced MRI

[c]Includes BS both with and without SPECT

[d]Includes both FDG-PET and FDG-PET/CT

IMWG guidelines recommend initial staging of patients with either multiple myeloma or monoclonal gammopathy of unknown significance (MGUS) but normal SS with (WB) MRI. This same technique also is recommended for the initial evaluation of patients with an apparently solitary plasmacytoma [34, 44].

FDG-PET has a higher sensitivity for myeloma bone lesions compared with SS [42], but FDG-PET appears to be less sensitive than MRI (particularly in the spine

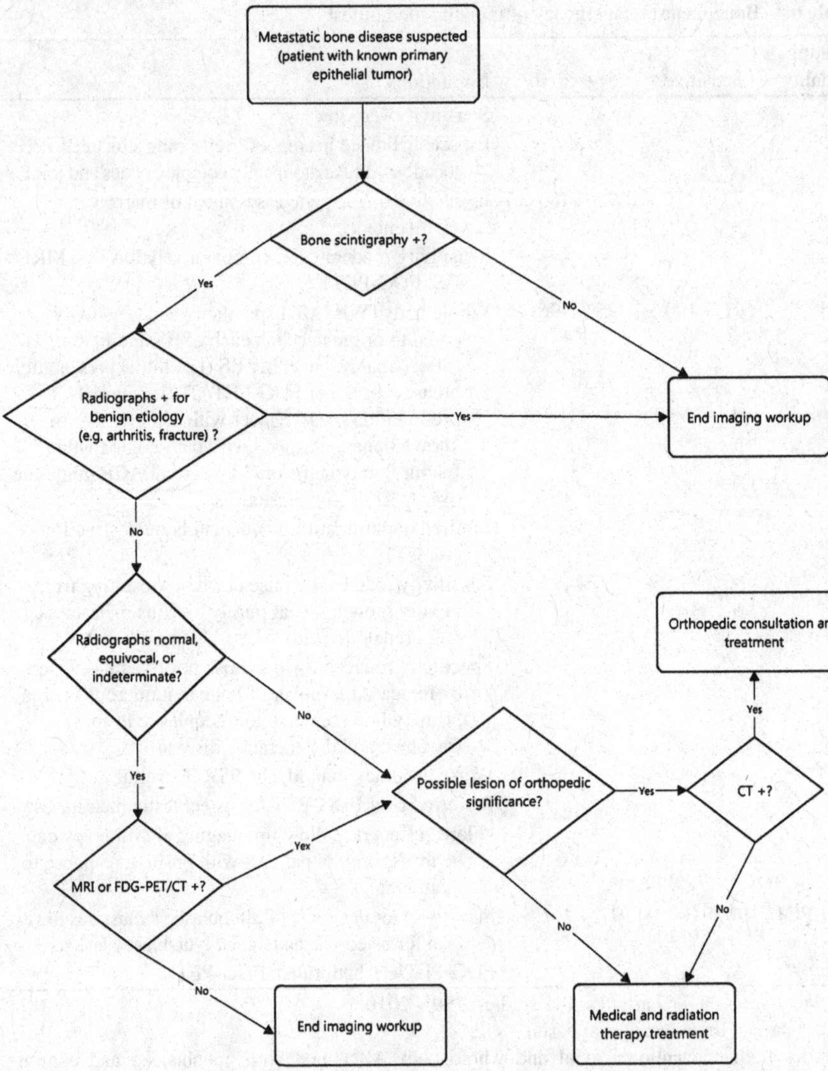

Fig. 6.8 Workup of metastatic bone disease

and pelvis), especially in cases of diffuse bone infiltration instead of localized lytic lesions [42, 45, 46]. Although more study is needed, at the current time MRI appears to be a better choice than FDG-PET for the initial staging of MM [42]. On the other hand, FDG-PET, with its ability to provide information about the physiologic activity of disease, may be preferable to MRI for follow-up imaging since treated lesions may still be evident on MR after therapy [45].

In summary, despite the limitations of SS and evidence in the literature of much higher sensitivity for more advanced imaging techniques such as (WB) MRI,

FDG-PET, and FDG-PET/CT, skeletal survey presently remains the gold standard in imaging workup of MM [34]. In addition, since according to current guidelines of the IMWG, only symptomatic MM patients receive treatment, skeletal survey remains the mainstay of radiological evaluation of myeloma patients (Table 6.5, Fig. 6.9).

All in all, radiographs form the lynch pin of accurate diagnosis of focal osseous lesions. They serve as the first line of imaging, except in a few specific clinical situations as described above. In cases where radiographs are non-diagnostic, in younger patients and in patients who have no history of epithelial neoplasm, MRI is usually the next study chosen to evaluate an osseous lesion [47]. On the other hand, if the lesion's appearance is consistent with a metastasis from an epithelial tumor, BS is usually the next study chosen in order to determine if there are other metastases elsewhere in the skeleton [12, 47]. Overall, CT is used less frequently than MRI, but it is the correct choice in selected circumstances: some specific entities, e.g., osteoid osteoma, certain anatomic locations, e.g., juxtacortical or location in a flat bone, to evaluate tumor matrix, i.e., osteoid, chondroid, and to evaluate if a lesion is of orthopedic significance [32].

Soft Tissue Lesions

Typically, patients present for evaluation of a soft tissue mass because they have noted a palpable lesion, a new localized asymmetry in the appearance of their body, or pain in a specific area. Sometimes clinicians may detect the masses or asymmetries on physical examination. Benign tumors of the soft tissues are overwhelmingly more common than malignant soft tissue tumors (100:1) [48], the most common being a lipoma.

While CR is typically the first examination to evaluate bone lesions, it has little utility for soft tissue masses other than occasionally to show evidence of fat or some calcification or ossification within a mass. More advanced imaging, particularly MRI, but also US and CT, is required to visualize and characterize soft tissue mass lesions [23].

MRI is the gold standard for evaluation of soft tissue masses, again because of its inherent soft tissue contrast resolution [23, 32, 39, 48, 49]. Because MRI can show bone marrow and cortical bone destruction, it readily depicts when a mass involves or arises from the marrow space to secondarily involve the adjacent soft tissues and vice versa.

In cases where a lesion is suspected on physical examination, MRI can confirm whether or not a lesion is actually present [39]. The technique can also distinguish between cystic and solid masses. MRI is the preferred imaging modality to evaluate spontaneous soft tissue hemorrhage in middle age and elderly adults as this is often a sign of an underlying neoplasm [23].

In the majority of cases, MRI findings will characterize the mass, what adjacent structures the mass involves and in some cases whether the mass is benign or

Table 6.5 Multiple myeloma: efficacy of imaging modalities

Imaging modality	Sensitivity	Advantages	Limitations
CR/Skeletal survey	80 %	Widely available Allows for screening evaluation entire body	Extended acquisition time (minimum 20 films) Limited evaluation of ribs, sternum, and scapula At least 30 % trabecular bone destruction needed for detection Gold standard inferior to each of FDG-PET, FDG-PET/CT, and MRI but still most common initial imaging study
CT		Helpful in evaluation of deep structures and assessment of atypical and irregular bones and joints, and complex joint anatomy (e.g., sternum, sternoclavicular joint, spine, pelvis) Precise anatomic localization of findings Depicts subtle, early bone cortex erosion	Insensitive, inadequate assessment of marrow involvement Lower sensitivity (vs. MRI, FDG-PET)
MRI (without IV contrast)		Excellent bone marrow evaluation Superb anatomic detail Sensitivity and specificity high	Inferior assessment of mineralized bone damage (vs. CT)
BS	50 % (35–60 %)	Widely available	Sensitivity very low (worst of any modality) High false negative rate due to rapidly growing, near purely osteolytic lesions (e.g., renal, thyroid)
FDG-PET	90 %	Allows for evaluation of entire body Physiologic information Most likely preferable to MRI for follow-up imaging, response to treatment, etc. (further studies needed)	Most likely more for problem solving instead of routine staging FDG-PET/CT more accurate than FDG-PET Good coregistration of physiological and anatomical information in hybrid FDG-PET/CT raises localization ability of imaging

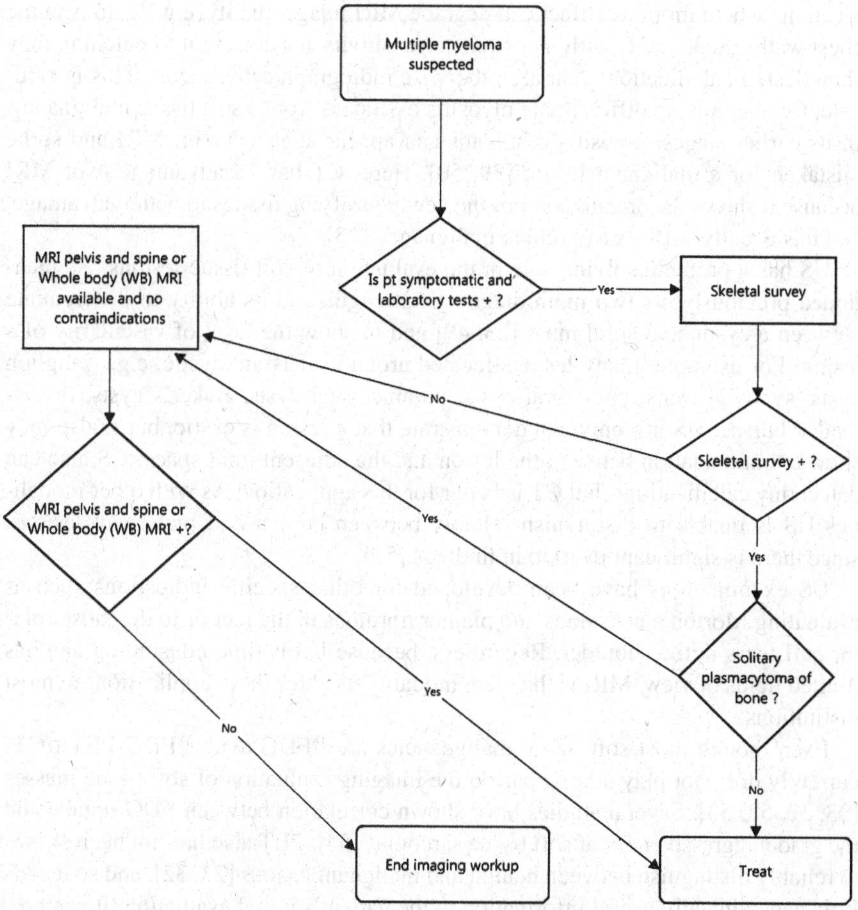

Fig. 6.9 Workup of multiple myeloma

malignant. Some lesions have a characteristic MRI appearance, permitting a confident diagnosis, e.g., various types of cysts, soft tissue hemangioma, lipoma, Morton's neuroma, plantar fibroma, elastofibroma, and fibrolipomatous hamartoma [39, 48, 49].

In the majority of cases, however, MRI findings will not yield a single diagnosis or sometimes even a confident determination that a lesion is benign [39, 48]. Because MRI can differentiate between necrotic/cystic and more viable, solid areas of a tumor, it may be used to direct where a lesion should be biopsied [23, 32].

Historically, CT was a front line imaging study for detection and characterization of soft tissue masses. As noted above, MRI has largely replaced CT in this capacity. In specific situations CT still has a role in evaluation of focal soft tissue lesions, for example to detect and characterize calcifications within a lesion or in anatomic locations where motion artifact can degrade MRI image quality, e.g., lesions in the chest wall [23, 32]. CT, with its exquisite sensitivity for detection of calcium, may show lesion calcifications that are otherwise radiographically occult. This is valuable, for example, to differentiate myositis ossificans from a soft tissue malignancy. In its earlier stages, myositis ossificans can appear aggressive on MRI and so be mistaken for a malignant lesion [39, 50]. Here, CT has an advantage over MRI because it shows the organization of the newly ossifying tissues to better advantage, and this usually suffices to exclude malignancy [23].

US has a problem solving role in the evaluation of soft tissue lesions. As mentioned previously, its two main diagnostic strengths are its ability to differentiate between a cystic and solid mass [23, 49] and to show the level of vascularity of a lesion. For example, many lesions located around joints are cystic, e.g., ganglion cysts, synovial cysts, paralabral cysts, parameniscal cysts, Baker's cysts, or distended bursae. US not only can demonstrate that a lesion is cystic, but it also may show communication between the lesion and the adjacent joint space. US also can detect tiny calcifications, but CT is better for this application. As with other modalities US is unable to distinguish reliably between benign and malignant lesions, since there is significant overlap in findings [51].

US examinations have been developed for other specific indications such as evaluating Morton's neuromas and plantar fibromas in the feet or to diagnose rotator cuff tears in the shoulder. Regardless, because US is time-consuming and has limited fields of view, MRI is the main modality used for these applications at most institutions.

Even though most soft tissue malignancies are ^{18}FDG avid, ^{18}FDG-PET (/CT) currently does not play a large part in the imaging evaluation of soft tissue masses [23, 32, 52, 53]. Several studies have shown correlation between FDG uptake and the grade/aggressiveness of soft tissue sarcomas [54]. PET also has not been shown to reliably distinguish between benign and malignant lesions [23, 32], and so it adds little new clinically useful information to the patient's initial evaluation. It can provide value, however, in directing tissue biopsy to more metabolically active portions of a lesion [13, 55]. PET imaging also is valuable to follow treated lesions since it displays a measure of metabolic activity in the former tumor bed [53].

As expected, BS has limited utility in the evaluation of soft tissue lesions. Only a small minority of lesions can be seen on BS, largely because most soft tissue lesions lack the osteoblastic activity that BS is designed to detect.

In summary, the detection and characterization of soft tissue lesions is usually not as straightforward as with primary bone tumors. In contrast to focal bone lesions, only a small percentage of soft tissue masses will be visible on CR. Regardless, CR is generally the initial diagnostic imaging study [48]. In selected cases, plain radiographs serve as a useful adjunct to more advanced imaging modalities [23]. MRI is the current gold standard for evaluation and diagnosis of soft tissues lesions, mainly because of its superb soft tissue contrast resolution [39, 49]. In certain circumstances, however, CT may be preferable to MRI [25]. PET may have greater importance in the future, but it needs additional vetting before it becomes a routine part of the imaging armamentarium [23, 49] (Fig. 6.10).

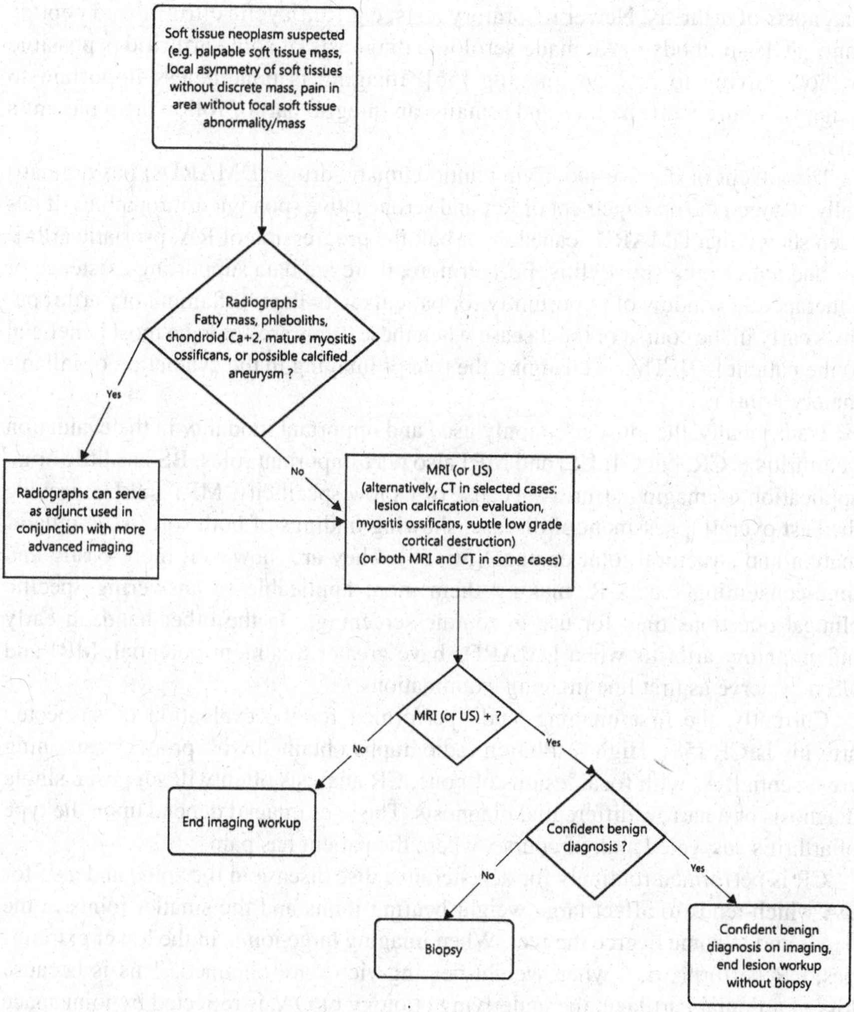

Fig. 6.10 Workup of primary soft tissue lesions

Arthritis

Although there are numerous well-known arthropathies, only three account for the vast majority of arthritis cases: osteoarthritis (OA), reflecting approximately 80 % of patients, rheumatoid arthritis (RA) and gout, each representing about 8 % of cases [13]. Regardless of the type of arthropathy, the initial evaluation of the patient is the same.

Clinical information including history, physical examination, symptoms, and laboratory data (serology, joint aspirate, etc.) plays an important role in the diagnosis of arthritis. Newer laboratory tests, e.g., anticyclic citrullinated peptide (anti-CCP) antibody, have made serologic diagnosis of some arthritides possible without having to rely on imaging [56]. Imaging is nonetheless important to diagnose many arthropathies and remains an integral part of following a patient's course.

The advent of disease-modifying antirheumatic drugs (DMARDs) has dramatically changed the management of RA and seronegative spondyloarthropathies. It has been shown that DMARDs can slow or halt the progression of RA, psoriatic arthritis, and ankylosing spondylitis. Furthermore, there are data supporting existence of a therapeutic window of opportunity for patients with these inflammatory arthropathies early in the course of the disease when these drugs are apt to be most beneficial to the patient [57]. This is changing the role of imaging in the evaluation of inflammatory arthritis.

Traditionally, the most commonly used and important modality in the evaluation of arthritis is CR, but CT, US, and MRI also play important roles. BS has little or no application to imaging arthritis because of its low specificity. MRI and US provide the best overall assessment of disease, showing findings of both soft tissue inflammation and structural joint damage [56, 58]. They are, however, more costly and time-consuming than CR, making them more applicable to answering specific clinical questions than for use in routine screening. On the other hand, in early inflammatory arthritis when DMARDs have greater treatment potential, MRI and US may serve as first line imaging examinations.

Currently, the first imaging study performed for the evaluation of suspected arthritis is CR [58]. High resolution radiographs obtained with proper positioning are essential. As with focal lesions of bone, CR analysis often will suggest a single diagnosis or a narrow differential diagnosis. The sites imaged depend upon the type of arthritis suspected and, of course, where the patient has pain.

CR is performed routinely for degenerative disc disease in the spine and also for OA which tends to affect large weight-bearing joints and the smaller joints in the hands and to some degree the feet. When imaging large joints in the lower extremities, CR performs best when weight-bearing views are obtained. This is because loss of articular cartilage, the underlying etiology of OA, is reflected by joint space narrowing on CR and this is best evaluated when the joints are under load.

During early stages of arthritis, radiographs do not correlate well with clinical measures such as pain and disability. This is related to the relative insensitivity of CR, and so it is not until the patient has progressed to later stages that radiographs correlate with functional outcome measures. In addition, CR rarely identifies synovitis, bursitis, and inflammatory soft tissues changes such as tenosynovitis that characterize the early phases of inflammatory arthritis [58].

Such findings are all easily seen on MRI and US. In addition, MRI can detect marrow edema which is the strongest predictor of future development and progression of erosions and subsequent loss of articular cartilage [56]. Synovitis and marrow edema, in particular, often precede and predict later bone erosions and the chondral loss that result in irreversible joint damage. As a result, MRI, and to a lesser extent, US are gaining popularity in evaluation of inflammatory arthropathies early in the course of disease [58].

CT is helpful in evaluating joints where anatomic complexity, joint orientation, or joint obscuration by adjacent structures limit the efficacy of radiographs, e.g., the sternoclavicular, temporomandibular, and sacroiliac joints. The main advantage and utility of CT is its ability to demonstrate cortical erosions, even those that are very small and subtle, and also to quantify total bone erosion volumes [59].

CT is at least equal to and possibly superior to MRI and US in erosion identification [58–60]. Unlike MRI, however, it cannot identify the bone marrow edema that precedes development of erosions, and it is also poor at detection of synovial proliferation and soft tissue inflammatory changes. Thus, CT is comparatively insensitive for detection of early arthritis, and so is rarely used in clinical practice except occasionally as a problem solving tool used in regions of difficult anatomy and some cases of septic arthritis and gout [58].

The sensitivity of US in detecting bone erosions is site-dependent, high in easily accessible joints but reduced in anatomically complicated joints [25, 58]. Where accessibility is optimal, US shows high agreement with MRI and possibly even CT at detection of bone erosions [58, 59]. Some studies suggest that US using color Doppler is more sensitive than MRI in showing the presence of synovitis and better in characterizing the synovitis by showing increased vascularity in inflamed tissue. As might be expected, joint effusions and synovitis which present clinically as periarticular soft tissue swelling are more easily identified using US than by physical examination [58]. Thus, given the importance of instituting DMARDs in a timely manner, US with its high sensitivity for identification of synovitis, bursitis, and inflammatory soft tissues changes has had an increasing role in early stage inflammatory arthropathies [58].

MRI can not only show erosions and joint space narrowing associated with inflammatory arthritis, but it also depicts both extra- and intra-articular soft tissue inflammatory changes early in the course of disease. As mentioned, not only does it show synovitis, but it also shows bone marrow edema that occurs in early disease [56]. This marrow edema histologically represents true osteitis consisting of active bone inflammation with cellular inflammatory infiltrates, but there is no free water making the term edema somewhat of a misnomer. Bone marrow "edema" on MRI predicts future erosions better than any other imaging finding [56]. Ultimately, the main goal of MRI is to identify precursor lesions before arthritis progresses to bone erosion, cartilage destruction, and joint structural damage [56]. Early imaging diagnosis of inflammatory arthritis will thus allow the clinician to institute prompt, effective treatment with DMARDs and so slow or even halt progression of the disease.

Regrettably, serologic testing, with the possible exception of anti-CCP antibody for RA, does not predict the future severity of an arthropathy [56]. This has led MRI to become a commonly used tool for the early diagnosis of clinically suspected undifferentiated inflammatory arthritis. The great disparity in cost and time of

Table 6.6 Inflammatory arthropathies: efficacy of imaging modalities for findings in early and late disease

Imaging modality	Early (joint effusion, synovitis, tenosynovitis)	Early (bone marrow edema)	Late (erosions)	Limitations
CR	+	–	++	Radiation exposure 2-D representation of 3-D information Very poor detecting early disease findings such as inflammatory soft tissue changes Sensitivity very low in demonstrating even findings of late disease (e.g.,) erosions-stage where therapeutic window for DMARDs has likely passed
US	+++++	–	++++	Operator-dependent Limited availability of well-trained, experienced, skillful MSK sonographers
CT	++	–	+++++	Radiation exposure Not adequate for detection of inflammatory soft tissue pathology and bone marrow findings of early disease
MRI	++++/+++++	+++++	++++	Not always (easily) available Expensive Long study length may result in image quality degraded by motion artifact (difficult for severely ill patients to remain in scanner for complete study) Nephrogenic systemic fibrosis (NSF) risk from IV gadolinium-based contrast agents (GBCAs) Less effective than CT in demonstrating early cortical bone erosion

acquisition between CR and MRI relative to the additional benefit provided by MRI militates against routine use of MRI over radiographs [58] (Table 6.6).

In summary, considerable advances have been made over the past decade in the application of advanced imaging techniques to diagnosing early RA and seronegative spondyloarthropathies, with an aim toward achieving improved clinical outcomes. Although CR is still the most frequently used imaging study for diagnosis of arthritis and is viewed as the "gold standard" [58] by the majority of the medical community, other more advanced imaging modalities are clearly more effective in detection of inflammatory changes in the soft tissues and identifying joint destruction. Radiographs have extremely low sensitivity in detection of non-osseous findings such as synovitis and tenosynovitis, and they are non-diagnostic in detection of bone marrow "edema"/osteitis, all findings of early disease in inflammatory

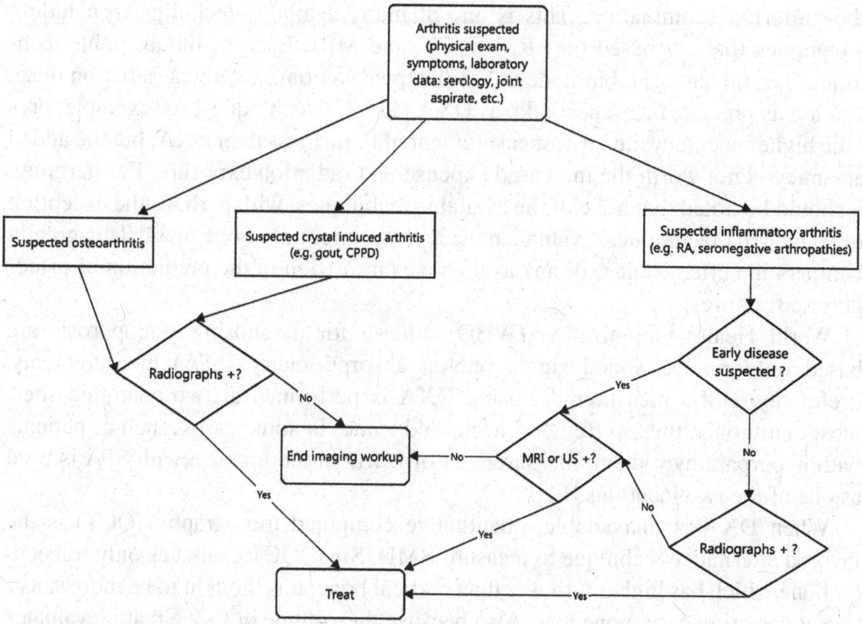

Fig. 6.11 Workup of inflammatory arthritis

arthropathies. US offers high sensitivity assessment, especially with regard to inflammatory soft tissue findings and for erosions related to joint damage. MRI and US are increasingly used in clinical practice with good benefit. CT, on the other hand, has a limited role in the clinical evaluation of arthritis [58]. The advent of DMARDs and hence the ability to arrest progression of disease has brought these more sophisticated studies to the fore (Fig. 6.11).

Metabolic

Osteoporosis

Osteoporosis is the loss of bone mass such that the skeleton becomes pathologically prone to fracture. Today, with people living longer lives, these fractures are a substantial source of morbidity and mortality. While previously the diagnosis of osteoporosis required occurrence of a fragility type fracture, we now are able to employ techniques that quantitatively determine bone mineral density (BMD). In the assessment of BMD, dual energy x-ray absorptiometry (DXA) is currently the preferred examination. This is one of many available techniques, including techniques that are based on CR, US, CT, and MRI. Each of the available techniques has advantages, but none are as inexpensive, have as low a radiation dose, and are as precise, i.e., repeatable, as DXA [61]. CT techniques, for example, provide higher accuracy, i.e., true measurement of bone mass than DXA, but the added accuracy is not worth the increased expense and radiation exposure. Furthermore, it should be noted that none of the available techniques, with perhaps the exception of some MRI techniques, evaluate bone architecture, only bone mass. This greatly hampers the effectiveness of any available examination in the prediction of osteoporotic fractures.

World Health Organization (WHO) criteria for diagnosing osteoporosis are based only on DXA and single photon absorptiometry (SPA) measurements. Preferably, BMD measurement using DXA is performed at two anatomic sites, most commonly, the hip (femoral neck) and spine. In some cases, such as patients with hyperparathyroidism, measurement of BMD in the forearm with SPA is used as one of the two locations [61].

When DXA is unavailable, quantitative computed tomography (QCT) is the favored alternative technique to measure BMD. Since QCT evaluates only trabecular bone which has higher turnover than cortical bone, it is thought to be more sensitive at detecting early bone loss. Also because the volume of tissue that it evaluates is directly measured and based on a projection like DXA, it is not prone to accuracy error from osteophytes and vascular calcifications in the path of the beam. Unfortunately, QCT cannot be used to diagnose osteoporosis based on the quantitative BMD value obtained, since it has never been validated for WHO criteria. However, through comparison of BMD values to a reference database for the technique, QCT can identify patients with low bone mass who are at risk for fracture [61].

Several other tests for BMD are also reliable in detection of those patients at risk for fracture. Techniques such as peripheral quantitative computed tomography (pQCT), peripheral quantitative ultrasound (pQUS), single X-ray absorptiometry (SXA) [62], and radiographic absorptiometry are less expensive and may be able to identify a larger percentage of the population at risk for osteoporotic fractures. Unlike DXA and QCT, these other technologies are not approved for following treatment [61].

BS, while it provides no information about BMD, is valuable in osteoporotic patients since it provides a whole body survey of the skeletal system for insufficiency fractures. This is particularly advantageous since osteoporosis-related fractures often occur in multiple locations, and some may be asymptomatic.

In conclusion, DXA is the current gold standard for measurement of BMD because it is both inexpensive and precise. Diagnosis of osteoporosis using WHO criteria is only possible with DXA and SPA. Many techniques, including MRI, pQCT, pQUS, SXA [62], and radiographic absorptiometry, are available to measure BMD, each with its own strengths and weaknesses (Tables 6.7 and 6.8).

Table 6.7 Imaging investigations for specific types of musculoskeletal pathology

Diagnosis	Imaging modality of choice in initial evaluation	Second most preferred imaging modality	Other imaging modalities (including role)	Additional points
Fracture	CR	MRI without contrast (occult acute traumatic fracture, stress fracture)	BS (diagnosis)	CR may take up to 7–10 days after injury to diagnose fracture
			CT (presurgical planning: e.g., complex fracture-dislocation)	MRI diagnosis within a few hours typically
				Usually takes 1–3 days after injury for high sensitivity fracture diagnosis on BS
Meniscal tear	MRI without contrast	CT arthrography (if MRI unavailable or contraindicated)		Conventional arthrography as last resort
Rotator cuff tear	MRI without contrast	US	CT arthrography (if MRI unavailable or contraindicated and US not offered)	MR arthrography preferred over conventional MRI without contrast for glenohumeral instability
				Conventional arthrography as last resort
Osteomyelitis	CR	MRI without and with IV contrast	MRI without IV contrast	CR sensitivity low
			BS	BS sensitivity high, specificity low
			Labeled WBC	Usually takes 2–3 days after start of infection for BS to diagnose
			BS + Labeled WBC	BS sensitivity increased by addition of labeled WBC study.
				Bone probe results may obviate need for imaging
			CT (assess pathologic fracture risk by identifying lesions of orthopedic significance)	Biopsy required in some cases (indeterminate, equivocal imaging)
Soft tissue abscess	CR	MRI without and with IV contrast	MRI without IV contrast	CR sensitivity low
		US	CT with IV contrast	US, MRI with IV contrast, and labeled WBC sensitivity and specificity high
			Labeled WBC	US and CT can guide aspiration

(continued)

Table 6.7 (continued)

Diagnosis	Imaging modality of choice in initial evaluation	Second most preferred imaging modality	Other imaging modalities (including role)	Additional points
Primary bone tumor	CR	Aggressive or indeterminate lesion on CR: BS (To determine if there is multifocal disease)		
		Thyroid cancer		
Bone metastases	CR (specific site clinically suspected)	CR (1 or more indeterminate or equivocal lesions on screening BS)	CT (assess pathologic fracture risk-identify lesions of orthopedic significance)	CR insensitive (at least 30 % bone destruction needed for detection)
	BS (screening for multifocal disease)	BS (CR normal)		BS sensitivity moderate to high, specificity moderate
	FDG-PET/CT	FDG-PET/CT (BS or CR normal)		Total body survey possible using BS, FDG-PET/CT, or WB MRI
	Whole body (WB) MRI	MRI (BS abnormal then CR normal, indeterminate or equivocal)		WB MRI specificity and sensitivity equal to or greater than each of BS and FDG-PET/CT separately, but in virtually all ACR appropriateness criteria clinical scenario variants these two modalities are favored over MRI
Multiple myeloma	Skeletal survey (if symptomatic), and laboratory tests abnormal	Whole body MRI MRI spine/pelvis if SS normal or with solitary plasmacytoma of bone	CT (assess pathologic fracture risk-identify lesions of orthopedic significance)	BS lacks sensitivity
Early rheumatoid arthritis	MRI without and with IV contrast US	MRI without and with IV contrast US	CT (erosions)	CR insensitive to identify findings of early disease (e.g., tenosynovitis, synovitis, bone marrow edema)
Established rheumatoid arthritis	CR	MRI without and with IV contrast US (if CR negative for RA, OA, gout, etc.)	CT (erosions)	CR sensitivity limited for findings of late disease, e.g., erosions

Table 6.8 2012 Medicare global reimbursement of various imaging modalities

Imaging modality	2012 Reimbursement ($)
CR	35
Skeletal survey	75
US limited (mass)	45
US complete (tendons, muscles, etc.)	130
CT (w/o, w/)	245–300
BS	275
BS (3 phase)	315
Labeled WBC study	375
MRI (w/o, w/ and w/o)	430–675
PET/CT	1,225

References

1. American College of Radiology. ACR Appropriateness Criteria®: Suspected spine trauma. Available at: http://www.acr.org/~/media/ACR/Documents/AppCriteria/Diagnostic/SuspectedSpineTrauma.pdf.
2. American College of Radiology. ACR Appropriateness Criteria®: Acute hand and wrist trauma. Available at: http://www.acr.org/~/media/ACR/Documents/AppCriteria/Diagnostic/AcuteHandandWristTrauma.pdf.
3. Rao N, Hrehorovich P, Mathew M. Acute osseous injury to the wrist. In: Pope TL, Bloem HL, Beltran J, Morrison WB, Wilson DJ, editors. Imaging of the musculoskeletal system. 1st ed. Philadelphia: Saunders Elsevier; 2008.
4. Mellado JM, Hualde AM, Albareda J, Llopis E. Acute osseous injury to the hip and proximal femur. In: Pope TL, Bloem HL, Beltran J, Morrison WB, Wilson DJ, editors. Imaging of the musculoskeletal system. 1st ed. Philadelphia: Saunders Elsevier; 2008.
5. Helms CA, Major NM, Anderson MW, Kaplan PA, Dussault R, editors. Osseous trauma. In: Musculoskeletal MRI. 2nd ed. Philadelphia: Saunders Elsevier; 2009. pp. 153–171.
6. Blankenbaker DG, Davis KW, Daffner RH. Cervical spine injuries. In: Pope TL, Bloem HL, Beltran J, Morrison WB, Wilson DJ, editors. Imaging of the musculoskeletal system. 1st ed. Philadelphia: Saunders Elsevier; 2008.
7. Llopis E, Higuera V, Aparisi P, Mellado JM, Aparisi F. Acute osseous injury to the pelvis and acetabulum. In: Pope TL, Bloem HL, Beltran J, Morrison WB, Wilson DJ, editors. Imaging of the musculoskeletal system. 1st ed. Philadelphia: Saunders Elsevier; 2008.
8. Zoga AC, Karasick D. Acute osseous injury to the knee. In: Pope TL, Bloem HL, Beltran J, Morrison WB, Wilson DJ, editors. Imaging of the musculoskeletal system. 1st ed. Philadelphia: Saunders Elsevier; 2008.
9. American College of Radiology. ACR Appropriateness Criteria®: Acute trauma to knee. Available at: http://www.acr.org/~/media/ACR/Documents/AppCriteria/Diagnostic/AcuteTraumaKnee.pdf.
10. Greaney RB, Gerber FH, Laughlin RL, et al. Distribution and natural history of stress fractures in U.S. Marine military recruits. Radiology. 1983;146:339–46.
11. Ahn JM, El-Khoury GY. Stress injury. In: Pope TL, Bloem HL, Beltran J, Morrison WB, Wilson DJ, editors. Imaging of the musculoskeletal system. 1st ed. Philadelphia: Saunders Elsevier; 2008.
12. American College of Radiology. ACR Appropriateness Criteria®: Metastatic bone disease. Available at: http://www.acr.org/~/media/ACR/Documents/AppCriteria/Diagnostic/MetastaticBoneDisease.pdf.

13. Reinus WR. Imaging approach to musculoskeletal infections. In: Bonakdarpour A, Reinus WR, Khurana JS, editors. Diagnostic imaging of musculoskeletal diseases: a systematic approach. 1st ed. New York: Springer; 2009.
14. Khan SHM, Bloem HL. Infection in the appendicular skeleton (including chronic osteomyelitis). In: Pope TL, Bloem HL, Beltran J, Morrison WB, Wilson DJ, editors. Imaging of the musculoskeletal system. 1st ed. Philadelphia: Saunders Elsevier; 2008.
15. Helms CA, Major NM, Anderson MW, Kaplan PA, Dussault R, editors. Musculoskeletal infections. In: Musculoskeletal MRI. 2nd ed. Philadelphia: Saunders Elsevier; 2009. pp. 92–110.
16. Resnick D. Osteomyelitis, septic arthritis, and soft tissue infection: mechanisms and situations. In: Resnick D, editor. Bone and Joint Imaging. 2nd ed. Philadelphia: W.B. Saunders; 1996. p. 649–73.
17. Morrison W, Ledermann HP. Diabetic pedal infection. In: Pope TL, Bloem HL, Beltran J, Morrison WB, Wilson DJ, editors. Imaging of the musculoskeletal system. 1st ed. Philadelphia: Saunders Elsevier; 2008.
18. Tumeh SS, Aliabadi P, Weissman BN, McNeil BJ. Disease activity in osteomyelitis: role of radiography. Radiology. 1987;165:781–4.
19. Morrison WB, Schweitzer ME, Bock GW, et al. Diagnosis of osteomyelitis: utility of fat-suppressed contrast-enhanced MR imaging. Radiology. 1993;189:251–7.
20. Ledermann HP, Schweitzer ME, Morrison WB. Nonenhancing tissue on MR imaging of pedal infection—characterization of necrotic tissues and associated limitations for diagnoses of osteomyelitis and abscess. American J Roengten. 2002;178:215–22.
21. Thrall JH, Ziessman HA, editors. Infection and inflammation. In: Nuclear medicine: the requisites. 1st ed. St. Louis: Mosby-Year Book; 1995.
22. Termaat MF, Raijmakers PG, Scholten HJ, et al. The accuracy of diagnostic imaging for the assessment of chronic osteomyelitis: a systematic review and meta-analysis. J Bone Joint Surg AM. 2005;87:2464–71.
23. American College of Radiology. ACR Appropriateness Criteria®: Soft tissue masses. Available at: http://www.acr.org/~/media/ACR/Documents/AppCriteria/Diagnostic/SoftTissueMasses.pdf.
24. Jelinek JS, Kransdorf MJ, Shmookler BM, Aboulafia AJ, Malawer MM. Liposarcoma of the extremities: MR and CT findings in the histologic subtypes. Radiology. 1993;186(2):455–9.
25. Tins B, Cassar-Pullicino V. Spinal infection. In: Pope TL, Bloem HL, Beltran J, Morrison WB, Wilson DJ, editors. Imaging of the musculoskeletal system. 1st ed. Philadelphia: Saunders Elsevier; 2008.
26. Wilson D, Atkins B. Soft tissue disease: cellulitis, pyomyositis, abscess, septic arthritis. In: Pope TL, Bloem HL, Beltran J, Morrison WB, Wilson DJ, editors. Imaging of the musculoskeletal system. 1st ed. Philadelphia: Saunders Elsevier; 2008.
27. Beaman F, Bancroft L. Complications of infection. In: Pope TL, Bloem HL, Beltran J, Morrison WB, Wilson DJ, editors. Imaging of the musculoskeletal system. 1st ed. Philadelphia: Saunders Elsevier; 2008.
28. Helms CA, Major NM, Anderson MW, Kaplan PA, Dussault R. Tendons and muscles. Musculoskeletal MRI. 2nd ed. Philadelphia: Saunders Elsevier; 2009. pp. 50–71.
29. Schweitzer M, Birnbaum M. Imaging of diabetes mellitus and neuropathic arthropathy: the diabetic foot. Imaging of degenerative and traumatic conditions, Section II, pp.146–165
30. Sundaram M, McLeod RA. MR imaging of tumor and tumorlike lesions of bone and soft tissue. Am J Roentgenol. 1990;155(4):817–24.
31. Miller TT. Bone Tumors and Tumorlike Conditions: Analysis with Conventional Radiography. Radiology. 2008;246:662–74.
32. Parsons III TW, Frink SJ, Campbell SE. Musculoskeletal Neoplasia: Helping the Orthopaedic Surgeon Establish the Diagnosis. Semin Musculoskelet Radiol. 2007;11(1):3–15.
33. Yang H, Liu T, Wang X, Xu Y, Deng S. Diagnosis of bone metastases: a meta-analysis comparing FDG-PET, CT, MRI and bone scintigraphy. Eur Radiol. 2011;21:2604–17.
34. Dimopoulos M, Terpos E, Comenzo RL, Tosi P, Beksac M, Sezer O, et al. International myeloma working group consensus statement and guidelines regarding the current role of

imaging techniques in the diagnosis and monitoring of multiple myeloma. Leukemia. 2009; 23:1545–56.
35. Parsons III TW, Filzen TW. Evaluation and staging of musculoskeletal neoplasia. Hand Clin. 2004;20:137–45.
36. Holder LE. Clinical radionuclide bone imaging. Radiology. 1990;176(3):607–14.
37. Kara G, Bozkurt MF, Ozcan PP, Caner B. Solitary rib lesions in bone scans of patients with breast carcinoma. Nucl Med Commun. 2003;24:887–92.
38. Helms CA, Major NM, Anderson MW, Kaplan PA, Schweitzer DR, Birnbaum M. Tumors. Musculoskeletal MRI. Philadelphia, PA: Saunders/Elsevier; 2009. p. 123–52.
39. Wu JS, Hochman MG. Soft-tissue tumors and tumorlike lesions: a systematic imaging approach. Radiology. 2009;253(2):297–316.
40. Peterson JJ, Kransdorf MJ, O'Connor MI. Diagnosis of occult bone metastases: positron emission tomography. Clin Orthop Relat Res. 2003;(415 Suppl): S120–8.
41. Fogelman I, Cook G, Israel O, Van der Wall H. Positron emission tomography and bone metastases. Semin Nucl Med. 2005;35:135–42.
42. Lammeren-Venema D, Regelink J, Riphagen I, Zweegman S, Hoekstra O, Zijlstra J. F-Fluorodeoxyglucose positron emission tomography in assessment of myeloma related bone disease: a systematic review. Cancer. 2012;118:1971–81.
43. Hanrahan C, Christensen C, Crim J. Current Concepts in the Evaluation of Multiple Myeloma with MR Imaging and FDG PET/CT. RadioGraphics. 2010;30:127–42.
44. Terpos E, Moulopoulos L, Dimopoulos M. Advances in Imaging and the Management of Myeloma Bone Disease. J Clin Oncol. 2011;29(14):1907–15.
45. Lütje S, de Rooy J, Croockewit S, Koedam E, Oyen W, Raymakers R. Role of radiography, MRI and FDG-PET/CT in diagnosing, staging and therapeutical evaluation of patients with multiple myeloma. Ann Hematol. 2009;88:1161–8.
46. Hillengass J, Neben K, Goldschmidt H. Current status and developments in diagnosis and therapy of multiple myeloma. J Cancer Res Clin Oncol. 2010;136:151–5.
47. American College of Radiology. ACR Appropriateness Criteria®: Primary bone tumors. Available at: http://www.acr.org/~/media/ACR/Documents/AppCriteria/Diagnostic/PrimaryBoneTumors.pdf.
48. Kransdorf MJ, Murphey MD. Radiologic Evaluation of Soft-Tissue Masses: A Current Perspective. AJR. 2000;175:575–87.
49. de Schepper A. Soft tissue tumors. In: Pope TL, Bloem HL, Beltran J, Morrison WB, Wilson DJ, editors. Imaging of the musculoskeletal system. 1st ed. Philadelphia: Saunders Elsevier; 2008.
50. Reinus WR. Systemic approach to arthropathies. In: Bonakdarpour A, Reinus WR, Khurana JS, editors. Diagnostic imaging of musculoskeletal diseases: a systematic approach. 1st ed. New York: Springer; 2009.
51. Griffith JF, Chan DPN, Kumta SM, et al. Does Doppler analysis of musculoskeletal soft-tissue tumors help predict tumor malignancy? Clin Radiol. 2004;59(4):369–75.
52. Kransdorf MJ, Meis JM. Extraskeletal osseous and cartilaginous tumors of the extremities. RadioGraphics. 1993;13:853–84.
53. Bredella M, Caputo G, Steinbach L. Value of FDG positron emission tomography in conjunction with MR imaging for evaluating therapy response in patients with musculoskeletal sarcomas. AJR. 2002;179:1145–50.
54. Bastiaannet E, Groen H, Jager PL, et al. The value of FDG-PET in the detection, grading and response to therapy of bone and soft tissue sarcomas; a systematic review and meta-analysis. Cancer Treat Rev. 2004;30:83–101.
55. Jadvar H, Gamie S, Ramanna L, Conti PS. Musculoskeletal system. Semin Nucl Med. 2004; 34:254–61.
56. Demertzis J, Rubin D. MR imaging assessment of inflammatory crystalline -induced, and infectious arthritides. Magn Reson Imaging Clin N Am. 2011;19:339–63.
57. Baillet A, Gaujoux-Viala C, Mouterde G, Pham T, Tebib J, Saraux A, et al. Comparison of the efficacy of sonography, magnetic resonance imaging and conventional radiography for the detection

of bone erosions in rheumatoid arthritis patients: a systematic review and meta-analysis. Rheumatology. 2011;50:1137–47.
58. Østergaard M, Pedersen S, Døhn U. Imaging in rheumatoid arthritis—status and recent advances for magnetic resonance imaging, ultrasonography, computed tomography and conventional radiography. Best Pract Res Clin Rheumatol. 22(6):1019–1044. Available at: http://www.sciencedirect.com.
59. Døhn U, Ejbjerg B, Hasselquist M, Narvestad E, Møller J, Thomsen H, Østergaard M. Detection of bone erosions in rheumatoid arthritis wrist joints with magnetic resonance imaging, computed tomography and radiography. Arthritis Res Ther. 2008;10:R25 (doi:10.1186/ar2378). Available at: http://arthritis-research.com/content/10/1/R25.
60. Døhn U, Ejbjerg B, Court-Payen M, Hasselquist M, Narvestad E, Szkudlarek M, Møller J, Thomsen H, Østergaard M. Are bone erosions detected by magnetic resonance imaging and ultrasonography true erosions? A comparison with computed tomography in rheumatoid arthritis metacarpophalangeal joints. Arthritis Res Ther. 2006;8:R110 (doi:10.1186/ar1995). Available at: http://arthritis-research.com/content/8/4/R110.
61. American College of Radiology. ACR Appropriateness Criteria®: Osteoporosis and Bone Mineral Density. Available at: http://www.acr.org/~/media/ACR/Documents/AppCriteria/Diagnostic/OsteoporosisAndBoneMineralDensity.pdf.
62. Kelly TL, Crane G, Baran DT. Single X-ray absorptiometry of the forearm: precision, correlation, and reference data. Calcif Tissue Int. 1994;54(3):212–8.

Chapter 7
Approach to Vascular Imaging

Vineet Chib

Introduction

Imaging of the vascular system, in theory, is straightforward. The choice of imaging modality depends on many factors, including the type of lesion suspected and its anatomic location. Ultrasound (US), computed tomographic angiography (CTA), magnetic resonance angiography (MRA), and conventional angiography comprise the main modalities used to image the vascular system. Each has its advantages and disadvantages. In general, conventional digital subtraction angiography (DSA) is the current gold standard for vascular evaluation. Because this modality requires catheterization of an artery, it is not without risk and should generally be reserved for emergencies, clinical questions where other modalities have proven inadequate or possible therapeutic interventions. Other modalities offer less invasive ways to evaluate the vascular system and provide information needed for diagnosis and treatment.

Ultrasound

Of the four modalities mentioned above, ultrasound is the least invasive. It allows imaging of superficial vessels without radiation or intravenous contrast administration. An ultrasound transducer, or probe, is placed on the skin and used to evaluate the underlying vasculature. Real time grey scale images and color Doppler imaging can be performed to evaluate the patency of vessels, evaluate changes in vessel flow patterns through the cardiac cycle and also the proximity of adjacent structures to vascular pathology.

V. Chib, M.D. (✉)
Department of Radiology, Temple University Hospital, 3401 N. Broad Street, Philadelphia, PA 19140, USA
e-mail: vineet.chib@tuhs.temple.edu

W.R. Reinus (ed.), *Clinician's Guide to Diagnostic Imaging*,
DOI 10.1007/978-1-4614-8769-2_7, © Springer Science+Business Media New York 2014

US has disadvantages, including difficulty imaging through adipose tissue, gas, and bone; limitations on its field of view; and dependence on the sonographer's skill. In general, US is well suited to evaluate lower extremity DVT. In obese patients, however, adipose tissue may prevent sufficient penetration and reflection of the sound waves, making diagnostic images difficult to obtain. The vasculature in the abdomen and the brain can be obscured by bowel gas and bone, respectively, again making imaging difficult, if not impossible.

Today, US is performed using hand held, real-time transducers. The volume of tissue visible at any given time is relatively limited compared with other techniques. Therefore, it is possible to overlook pathology even when a scan has been performed carefully. Finally, ultrasound is dependent on the skill of the person performing the study. Although US images are interpreted by a radiologist, a sonographer performs the initial scan. Because of the limited field of view and the freehand nature of scanning, the quality of US images is influenced heavily by the experience and training of the sonographer. It is then up to the radiologist to determine whether or not additional images are required or if he should scan the patient personally.

CT Angiography

Multidetector computed tomography (CT) with contrast administration is another common way to evaluate vascular structures. It is more invasive than ultrasound, requiring intravenous access and administration of iodinated contrast. In addition, CT uses ionizing radiation. Imaging after intravenous contrast injection must be timed properly to obtain opacification of the desired vessels. Arterial phase imaging requires a rapid rate of intravenous contrast administration as well as bolus tracking—repeated imaging with a detector over a vessel—to ensure the arterial system is enhanced properly. Similarly, enhancement of the venous system requires appropriate timing of image acquisition but this is not as sensitive to timing as arterial imaging.

As with all intravenously contrast injected CT scans, a small percentage of patients will have an allergic reaction to the contrast material. This reaction can range from benign urticaria to full blown anaphylaxis with cardiorespiratory collapse. Fortunately, the latter is uncommon.

Benefits of CT angiography include ease of accessibility, with multidetector CT (MDCT) available in most hospitals and outpatient centers. CTA generally is performed using standard protocols which limit operator dependence. CTA allows clear anatomic evaluation not only of the vessels, but also of adjacent structures

Magnetic Resonance Angiography

MRA uses magnetic resonance imaging (MRI) techniques to generate images of the flowing blood through a vessel and thus shows the intimal walls of the vessel in relief. Images can be obtained either with or without injected intravenous contrast media.

MRI takes advantage of the inherent molecular differences among different types of tissue to generate the images. In general, two different techniques are available to obtain images without contrast, phase contrast imaging, and time of flight imaging. The former relies on the difference in signal of protons in stationary and mobile tissue. The latter relies on the protons flowing into the imaged slice having no out of plane magnetization at the time of image acquisition. Each of these techniques is limited by various technical issues that determine where they may be used. 3D contrast-enhanced MRA is performed with an intravenous injection of gadolinium-based contrast agent and generally provides higher quality images than both non-contrast techniques.

MRA uses no radiation. Radio frequency energy is deposited in the tissues with MRI, but thus far, no significant health risks have been identified related to this. Furthermore, MR contrast agents are of a different class than the iodinated agents used with CTA and conventional angiography. Patients with allergy to the latter have no crossover with MR contrast. In fact, true allergic reactions to gadolinium-based MR contrast agents are rare. So MRA can be useful in patients with a known iodinated contrast allergy.

Nonetheless, MRA has significant limitations, including high expense, the relatively long time required for image acquisition, and the risk of nephrogenic systemic fibrosis (NSF). NSF is a rare syndrome believed to be related to gadolinium contrast exposure, primarily in patients with low glomerular filtration rates either from acute or chronic renal failure. Patients develop fibrosis of skin, joints, and internal organs (See Chap. 1 for further discussion). Recognition of NSF has limited the use of MRA as an alternative to CTA in patients with limited renal function.

Conventional Angiography

Conventional angiography, also called DSA and catheter-directed angiography, directly visualizes the target vessels and so is the gold standard of vascular imaging. Using this technique, a catheter is placed directly into the vessel and imaged by injecting iodinated contrast. In many cases, because the catheter is present in the vessel, pathology can be both diagnosed and treated during the same procedure.

Even so, this technique also has disadvantages. It is the most invasive of all techniques used to evaluate the vasculature. There are risks to performing a procedure including bleeding, vessel injury, inducing thrombosis within a small vessel, creating an embolic thrombus and, of course, contrast-induced nephropathy. Patients who are on blood thinners are at increased risk of bleeding when undergoing DSA. Access into the vascular system in patients with severe atherosclerotic disease may be precluded if the common femoral artery, the entry vessel of choice, is heavily calcified or occluded. In these instances, a radial or brachial artery approach could be considered. Iodinated contrast material is used for this procedure, and as with CTA this places patients at risk for allergic contrast reaction and contrast-induced nephropathy. It should be mentioned, however, that for unknown reasons, patients who receive intra-arterial contrast are at much lower risk for allergic contrast reactions than those who receive intravenous contrast.

Head/Neck Vascular Imaging

Carotid Artery Narrowing

Carotid artery atherosclerotic disease is a major preventable cause of stroke [1]. Imaging is undertaken when there are clinical indications, e.g., carotid bruit or transient ischemic attack, indicating that a patient may have carotid stenosis or a build-up of atherosclerotic plaque. The mainstay of carotid imaging is noninvasive duplex ultrasound. This procedure has become accepted widely as the first test of choice for imaging carotid stenosis in a patient with clinical risk factors. CTA and MRA may also be considered but have the disadvantages of cost, contrast, and radiation exposure. These tests are generally reserved for patients in whom ultrasound is equivocal or non-diagnostic.

Carotid Artery or Vertebral Artery Dissection

In a setting of trauma, carotid or vertebral artery dissection may be suspected when a patient has head or neck pain and neurologic symptoms such as dysarthria, weakness, ataxia, or scotoma. Cross-sectional imaging, either with CTA or MRA, has become the standard imaging technique because of its noninvasive nature and widespread availability [2]. Conventional angiography is generally reserved for cases where noninvasive methods are not diagnostic.

Internal Jugular Vein Thrombosis

Internal jugular vein thrombosis occurs in a number of settings. Patients with a history of head and neck infections, recent surgery, indwelling catheters, and/or drug use are at risk for thrombosing their Jugular vein. Propagation of thrombus including pulmonary embolism is associated with internal jugular vein thrombosis. Because of the morbidity and mortality associated with jugular thrombosis, diagnosis is important [3]. Here again, duplex ultrasonography is the first-line diagnostic test because it is readily available, safe, can be performed at the bedside if necessary, and is noninvasive. CTA and MRA are used as second-line tests when ultrasound is non-diagnostic.

Upper Extremity Deep Venous Thrombosis

Other than in dialysis patients, upper extremity deep venous thrombosis (DVT) is uncommon. It is associated with significant morbidity and mortality because of risk of pulmonary embolism, loss of venous access, and post-thrombotic syndrome [4]. Two forms of upper extremity DVT are described: Paget von Schrotter or effort thrombosis and secondary thrombosis. In effort thrombosis, a chronic compression at the thoracic inlet or outlet resulting from musculoskeletal structures in the costoclavicular space causes slow venous return and ultimately thrombosis in the veins of the extremity. Secondary thrombosis usually is caused by either hypercoagulable states or indwelling catheters. Color flow duplex imaging diagnoses upper extremity venous thrombosis with 78–100 % sensitivity and 82–100 % specificity making it the first-line study [5]. Diagnosis with duplex ultrasound can be limited by the overlying clavicle. In equivocal cases, catheter-directed venogram can be helpful both for diagnosis and treatment.

Arterial Vasculidities

Vasculidities comprise a rare group of diseases generally characterized by vascular inflammation and luminal occlusion. If untreated, vasculitis can lead to aneurysm formation, rupture of vessel, vessel stenosis or occlusion, and end organ infarction. Vasculidities are commonly categorized by the size of the vessel affected. Large vessel vasculidities include Behçet's syndrome, polymyalgia rheumatica, Takayasu's arteritis, and temporal arteritis. Medium-sized vessel vasculidities include Buerger's disease, Kawasaki disease, and polyarteritis nodosa. Small vessel vasculidities include Churg–Strauss syndrome, cutaneous vasculitis, Henoch–Schönlein purpura, microscopic polyangiitis, and Wegener's granulomatosis. Because of the large range of vessels affected by different forms of vasculitis, symptoms can be varied.

Diagnosis is commonly suggested by laboratory tests that show signs of inflammation such as erythrocyte sedimentation rate (ESR), C reactive protein (CRP), elevated white blood cell count, or eosinophilia. Organ-specific lab tests may also be abnormal if the specific end organ is affected by the vasculitis. Typically, biopsy of the affected organ will make the definitive diagnosis. Angiography can demonstrate characteristic findings that aid in the diagnosis of particular vasculidities.

Suppression of the inflammation mediated by the immune system using steroids is the mainstay of treatment. In cases of infection, antibiotics are prescribed. In acute vasculitis, the organ affected may require supportive treatment to improve function. Ultrasound is the most readily available, noninvasive way to evaluate for arterial stenosis or occlusion, the side effect of vasculitis. Imaging of central vascular structures can be limited with ultrasound as discussed earlier. CT angiography allows for evaluation of central vasculature as well as anatomy of adjacent structures. MRA can also be used to characterize vessel stenosis and occlusion. Conventional angiography is considered the gold standard for the diagnosis of vessel abnormalities and has the advantage of allowing for possible intervention.

Dialysis Access

Dialysis fistulas or grafts create a connection between the arterial and venous system. These create a conduit large enough to allow blood to be withdrawn from the body, filtered in a dialysis machine and then returned to the body. Dialysis fistulas tend to thrombose. In fact, patients with dialysis fistulas have a primary patency rate of approximately 35 % at 2 years after fistula creation [6]. One of the most common causes of hospital admission in the dialysis patients is fistual access problems making fistula patency maintenance an important part of renal failure patient management [7].

As most patients receive dialysis treatments between two and five times weekly, early assessment of fistula malfunction can be made by the dialysis center staff. Such evaluation includes physical examination for fistula pulsatility or thrill, suboptimal flow during dialysis, high pressures generated on the dialysis machine, or edema of the extremity. These indirect signs of fistula malfunction can be further evaluated noninvasively with ultrasound. No contrast media is required, reducing the risk of contrast reaction and further reducing renal function. US has no risk of injuring the fistula, and it provides information about the fistula's anatomy and flow. One drawback is US poorly visualizes veins more axial or central to the fistula. These often stenose and are responsible for fistula malfunction. A fistulagram, cannulation of the fistula with direct injection of intravenous contrast to opacify the fistula, is a more invasive way of assessing the fistula but allows better visualization of the central venous circulation. Direct fistula access also allows therapeutic intervention if an abnormality is identified.

Lower Extremity Deep Venous Thrombosis

The lower extremity is the most common location of DVT and the cause of 90 % of acute pulmonary emboli in the United States [8]. Therefore, diagnosis is very important. Underlying conditions predisposing a patient to DVT include venous stasis, injury to vessel walls, and hypercoagulable states. As with other forms of DVT, duplex US is the first-line imaging study because of its ready availability, ability to be performed portably, and lack of IV contrast and radiation. In the past, venography was the first-line examination. This test requires catheterization of a foot vein and injection of iodinated contrast followed by imaging using digital subtraction techniques. Venography, for the most part, has been replaced by ultrasound, but is still used in patients where ultrasound faces technical limitations, i.e., obese patients and patients with marked lower extremity edema. Venography also has a role as a second-line study when US studies are equivocal.

Peripheral Vascular Disease

Peripheral vascular disease (PVD), also known as peripheral artery occlusive disease, is most commonly caused by atherosclerosis and affects 12–14 % of patients in the general population and 20 % of patients over 70 [9]. In other words, PVD results from the same causes as coronary artery disease and cerebrovascular disease. Patients with PVD suffer significant debility and pain from claudication and are at increased risk of peripheral gangrene and limb loss caused by lack of blood flow related to vessel stenosis and occlusion. The initial diagnosis of PVD is made with ankle-brachial index (ABI) measurements that evaluate the ratio of upper to lower extremity arterial blood flow. If ABIs are abnormal, segmental Doppler pressures and pulse volume recordings can help localize levels of stenosis or occlusion. Cross-sectional angiography with CTA or MRA can be further used to visualize the degree and level of stenoses and occlusions. Today, conventional angiography is generally reserved for possible intervention such as angioplasty or stent placement.

Abdominal Vasculature

Mesenteric Ischemia

Mesenteric ischemia is caused by acutely or chronically decreased blood supply to the intestines. Both arterial and venous disease may cause mesenteric ischemia. On the arterial side, arterial stenosis, emboli, and thrombus cause acute mesenteric ischemia. At times ischemia also can result from non-occlusive disease as in cases of diminished blood volume related to hypervolemia.

Multiple studies have shown that CTA has sensitivity between 96 and 100 % and specificity between 89 and 94 % for the evaluation of mesenteric ischemia [10]. CTA provides information about the vessels, the bowel, and other abdominal organs. As a result CTA has largely replaced conventional angiography, once considered the gold standard in the evaluation of this disease. On the other hand, conventional angiography, by virtue of having a catheter directly in the arterial system, provides a therapeutic option including intra-arterial thrombolysis and vasodilator administration.

Gastrointestinal Hemorrhage

Clinically, gastrointestinal (GI) hemorrhage can be divided into gastric, upper, and lower intestinal sources of bleeding. Although most cases resolve with supportive measures, approximately 7 % of patients admitted with GI bleeding die during their hospitalization [11]. Endoscopic direct visualization of the bleeding source is the preferred method of diagnosis for upper GI hemorrhage. Lower GI bleeding is usually approached either using a nuclear medicine study such as a tagged red blood cell study or using proctoscopy or colonoscopy. In cases where endoscopy or nuclear studies fail to locate the source of bleeding, angiography should be performed [12]. It permits both localization of the source of hemorrhage and the possibility of embolizing the bleeding vessel to arrest the hemorrhage.

Abdominal Aortic Aneurysm/Dissection

Abdominal aortic aneurysm (AAA) has a prevalence of approximately 1–2 % of the population [13]. Ruptured AAA is the thirteenth leading cause of death in the United States [14]. As the diameter of the AAA increases, so does the risk of rupture. In general, aneurysms over 5.5 cm in size require treatment because of the high risk of mortality from rupture relative to the risk of surgery [15].

Abdominal ultrasound is an inexpensive and effective method to screen for suspected abdominal AAA. CTA of the aorta currently is the study of choice for evaluation of known AAA. Additionally, imaging of the thorax should be considered for patients in whom the thoracic aorta has not been evaluated. Patients who have had endograft treatment of AAA should also be screened with CTA to evaluate for endoleak, i.e., leaks around the stent. Catheter-directed angiogram should be reserved for cases where intra-arterial treatment of an AAA or of a resulting endoleak is planned.

Pelvic Congestion Syndrome

Pelvic congestion syndrome is a common but underdiagnosed cause of pelvic pain [16]. Dilated, tortuous congested pelvic veins with retrograde flow of blood through incompetent valves cause dull pelvic pain, pressure, and heaviness in patients with this disease [16]. Transvaginal ultrasound with color Doppler and Doppler spectral analysis can identify pelvic varices and thus be used to diagnose pelvic congestion. MRI can also be used although is not as cost effective as ultrasound and may not be as well tolerated by claustrophobic patients.

Varicocele

A varicocele is dilation of the pampiniform venous plexus of veins caused by absent or incompetent valves in the internal spermatic vein. Approximately 40 % of men being treated in infertility clinics have a varicocele [17], making varicoceles a major cause of male infertility. They cause poor sperm and decreased semen production. Patients may also complain of scrotal pain or heaviness. Diagnosis is often made on clinical exam in which case ultrasound can be used to confirm the diagnosis. Ultrasound also can diagnose varicoceles not identified on clinical exam [18]. Surgical repair of varicocele either can be performed in the outpatient setting or treated with percutaneous intravenous embolization to occlude the varicocele's venous supply.

Thoracic Vasculature

Superior Vena Cava Syndrome

Superior vena cava (SVC) syndrome results from obstruction of blood flow through the SVC. It most commonly presents with dyspnea but it may cause other symptoms including head and neck swelling (sometimes massive), chest pain, distorted vision, stridor, and headache. Many patients can be diagnosed on the basis of clinical symptoms alone. Most patients will have an abnormal chest X-ray. Indwelling central intravascular catheters are the most common benign cause of SVC syndrome [19]. Tumor invasion or extrinsic compression of the SVC is the most common malignant cause. Regardless, SVC syndrome should be considered a medical emergency. CT with contrast can determine whether extrinsic compression or thrombus is the cause of the obstruction. Direct contrast venogram is the most conclusive test to evaluate SVC syndrome and has the benefit of allowing venous access for treatment of the thrombus with either an endovascular stent or intravenous lysis. Radiation therapy has been the standard treatment for malignant SVC syndrome.

Thoracic Aortic Aneurysm/Dissection

Thoracic aortic aneurysm—focal aneurismal dilatation of the thoracic aorta—is the most common thoracic aortic disease requiring surgical intervention. Surgery is the treatment of choice for thoracic aneurysms that are 6 cm or greater in diameter.

Aortic dissection results from a tear in the intima or inner most layer of the aorta that allows blood to pass through the media into the adventitia or the outermost layer of the aorta. Blood rapidly accumulates and expands the outer adventitia of the aorta, putting the patient at risk for aortic rupture. Identification of the point of dissection as well as luminal diameter is key in determining treatment. Classically, dissection has been characterized by location as Stanford type A or type B dissections. Type A dissections involve the ascending aorta and arch proximal to the brachiocephalic artery origin. They are considered surgical emergencies because of the potential for extension proximally to the aortic valve, coronary arteries, or distally up into the carotid and vertebral arteries. Type B dissection involves the descending aorta or arch without ascending aorta involvement. These are dissections that are usually treaded medically [20].

CTA is the diagnostic modality of choice for evaluation of thoracic aortic dissection. CTA should include non-contrast imaging to evaluate for acute intramural hematoma as well as contrast imaging to visualize the dissection itself. CTA has largely replaced catheter-directed angiography because it has accuracy approaching 100 % and is less invasive, quicker, and generally available [21, 22].

Pulmonary Embolism

Pulmonary embolism is most commonly caused by DVT, but embolism can arise from other sites or from intravenous injection of drugs. In addition, emboli need not consist of hematologic thrombus but instead may be septic emboli from intravascular boli of bacteria, fat emboli from long bone trauma and in rare cases tumor thrombus. As with aortography, catheter-directed pulmonary angiography largely has been replaced by CTA which has become the standard for diagnosis of pulmonary embolism [23]. Nuclear medicine VQ scan is reserved for patients with contrast allergy or elevated creatinine who cannot undergo a CTA.

Percutaneous Biopsy

Imaging-directed percutaneous biopsy allows direct tissue sampling and pathologic diagnosis without the risks of surgery and anesthesia that are associated with open biopsy. Because percutaneous techniques are minimally invasive, they require little recovery time and so shorten hospital stays. Many locations within the body are amenable to image-guided percutaneous biopsy including thyroid, liver, pancreas, lung, and kidney.

Determining if a patient is a candidate for percutaneous biopsy is at the discretion of the physician performing the procedure. Review of diagnostic images is necessary to identify a safe percutaneous route into the lesion. Other considerations include the size of the lesion from which tissue sampling is requested. Critical structures such as the heart or pulmonary vessels located in proximity to a target lesion may preclude percutaneous biopsy, e.g., a lung nodule near the aorta or a thyroid mass near the carotid artery. If sedation is planned, the patient history should be reviewed for conditions such as obstructive sleep apnea. Blood thinning medications such as aspirin, Coumadin, or Lovenox, need to be held for several days prior to biopsy to reduce the risk of bleeding. Some patients may have conditions or devices like drug-eluting cardiac stents that preclude stopping aspirin or Plavix prior to biopsy. In these cases, a careful evaluation of the risks and benefits of the procedure must be weighed.

Conclusion

Imaging of the vascular system is theoretically straightforward. With current technology, diagnosis for many diseases can be made with noninvasive imaging techniques resulting in lower complication rates for patients. CTA is one of the most commonly used studies to evaluate vasculature of all body parts, given its availability and relative independence of operator error. However, ultrasound and MRA are also valuable tools in evaluation of the vasculature. Generally, catheter-directed angiography is reserved for situations in which noninvasive testing is equivocal or intervention is planned.

References

1. U-King-Im JM, Young V, Gillard JH. Carotid artery imaging in the diagnosis and management of patients at risk of stroke. Lancet Neurol. 2009;8(6):569–80.
2. Rodallec MH, Marteau V, Gerber S, Desmottes L, Zins M. Craniocervical arterial dissection: spectrum of imaging findings and differential diagnosis. Radiographics. 2008;28(6):1711–28.
3. Sheikh MA, Topoulos AP, Deitcher SR. Isolated internal jugular vein thrombosis: risk factors and natural history. Vasc Med. 2002;7(3):177–9.
4. Sajid MS, Ahmed N, Desai M, Baker D, Hamilton G. Upper limb deep vein thrombosis: a literature review to streamline the protocol for management. Acta Haematol. 2007;118(1):10–8.
5. Gaitini D, Beck-Razi N, Haim N, Brenner BJ. Prevalence of upper extremity deep venous thrombosis diagnosed by color Doppler duplex sonography in cancer patients with central venous catheters. J Ultrasound Med. 2006;25(10):1297–303.
6. Field M, MacNamara K, Bailey G, Jaipersad A, Morgan RH, Pherwani AD. Primary patency rates of AV fistulas and the effect of patient variables. J Vasc Access. 2008;9(1):45–50.
7. Carlson DM, Duncan DA, Naessens JM, Johnson WJ. Hospitalization in dialysis patients. Mayo Clin Proc. 1984;59(11):769–75.
8. Hull RD, Raskob GE, Hirsh J. Prophylaxis of venous thromboembolism: an overview. Chest. 1986;89:374S–83.
9. Shammas NW. Epidemiology, classification, and modifiable risk factors of peripheral arterial disease. Vasc Health Risk Manag. 2007;3(2):229–34.
10. Kirkpatrick ID, Kroeker MA, Greenberg HM. Biphasic CT with mesenteric CT angiography in the evaluation of acute mesenteric ischemia: initial experience. Radiology. 2003;229(1):91–8.
11. Palmer K, Nairn M. Guideline Development, Group (2008-10-10). Management of acute gastrointestinal blood loss: summary of SIGN guidelines. BMJ. 2008;337:a1832.
12. Schenker MP, Majdalany BS, Funaki BS, et al.; and Expert Panel on Vascular Imaging and Interventional Radiology. ACR Appropriateness Criteria® upper gastrointestinal bleeding. Reston (VA): American College of Radiology (ACR); 2010.
13. Upchurch Jr GR, Schaub TA. Abdominal aortic aneurysm. Am Fam Physician. 2006;73(7): 1198–204.
14. Kochanek KD, Smith BL. Deaths: preliminary data for 2002. Natl Vital Stat Rep. 2004 Feb 11;52(13):1–47.
15. Ernst CB. Abdominal aortic aneurysm. N Engl J Med. 1993;328:1167–72.
16. Kuligowska K, Deeds L. Pelvic pain: overlooked and underdiagnosed gynecologic conditions. Radiographics. 2005;25:3–20.
17. Gat Y, Bachar GN, Zukerman Z, Belenky A, Gornish M. Varicocele: a bilateral disease. Fertil Steril. 2004;81(2):424–9.
18. Chiou RK, Anderson JC, Wobig RK, Rosinsky DE, Matamoros Jr A, Chen WS, et al. Color Doppler ultrasound criteria to diagnose varicoceles: correlation of a new scoring system with physical examination. Urology. 1997 Dec;50(6):953–6.
19. Rice TW, Rodriguez RM, Light RW. The superior vena cava syndrome: clinical characteristics and evolving etiology. Medicine (Baltimore). 2006;85(1):37–42.
20. Nienbaber CA, Eagle KA. Aortic dissection: new frontiers in diagnosis and management. Circulation. 2003;108:628–35.
21. Nienaber CA, Kische S, Skriabina V, Ince H. Noninvasive imaging approaches to evaluate the patient with known or suspected aortic disease. Circ Cardiovasc Imaging. 2009;2:499–506.

22. Shiga T, Wajima Z, Apfel CC, Inoue T, Ohe Y. Diagnostic accuracy of transesophageal echocardiography, helical computed tomography, and magnetic resonance imaging for suspected thoracic aortic dissection: systematic review and meta-analysis. Arch Intern Med. 2006;166(13):1350–6.
23. Bettmann MA, Lyders EM, Yucel EK, et al. American College of Radiology appropriateness criteria acute chest pain—suspected pulmonary embolism. Reston, VA: American College of Radiology (ACR); 2011. p. 7.

Index

W.R. Reinus (ed.), *Clinician's Guide to Diagnostic Imaging*,
DOI 10.1007/978-1-4614-8769-2, © Springer Science+Business Media New York 2014